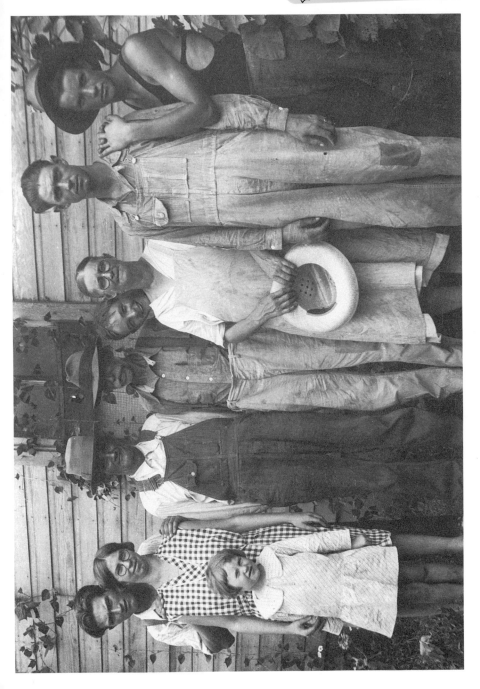

GRANDMA CHERRY'S SPOON

A Story of Tuberculosis

GRANDMA CHERRY'S SPOON

A Story of Tuberculosis

Marjorie McVicker Sutcliffe

with Judy Sutcliffe

GERONIMA PRESS
Santa Barbara, California

Photos of Grandma Cherry and family in Crocker, Missouri, 1930, were
taken by Marjorie McVicker and printed from the original negatives by
her daughter Juana Reynard in 1985. Endpaper photo shows author's
brother John Joseph and father, John William McVicker, at left,
amid cousins. Juana Reynard took the back cover
photo of the author in 1989.

Geronima Press
2216 Cliff Drive
Santa Barbara, CA 93109

Phone orders (VISA/Mastercard): 805/966-7563

CONTENTS

Foreword

Introduction

DEDICATED to all the medical professionals who nearly succeeded in eradicating tuberculosis from planet earth. May they never give up.

AND TO the good people of Hays, Kansas.

Marjorie McVicker Sutcliffe's reminiscences of her family's and her personal struggles with tuberculosis in the first half of this century will be of great interest to those who are concerned about the lives and deaths of earlier generations. However, her story has a much more immediate contemporary relevance than is at first apparent. California and much of the rest of the U.S. face a resurgence of tuberculosis, at a time when many thought that it could be eliminated from the nation within the next generation.

Despite effective and powerful drugs to treat the disease and well-honed control programs to identify those who become infected, cases are multiplying in many communities. As in the past, poverty and ignorance help its spread. Migrants from less fortunate lands where the disease is still common are one major source of cases coming into communities. Desperate overcrowding in inadequate housing encourages its spread. Added to this is the parallel epidemic of HIV infection leading to AIDS. Those infected with HIV are highly susceptible both to primary infection or secondary breakdown of latent infection with the tubercle bacillus. Tuberculosis is becoming the leading cause of death in AIDS patients in some parts of the world. The association of these diseases is a major factor in the increasing case loads of TB in some areas of the U.S. To compound our problems, some of the bacteria, particularly from Asia, have become resistant to some or most of the drugs that we have. Outbreaks caused by resistant strains have been reported from Florida, Texas and a California prison.

We are fortunate that nowadays, with our modern drugs, the prolonged rest and isolation for control of the disease are usually no longer needed. Resumption of work within a few weeks of starting a 6–12 month course of treatment is usual and safe. Tuberculosis control programs can now focus on contact identification and treatment to prevent further generations of infection, coupled with tracking sources of new cases. Given adequate government support, tuberculosis can be brought back under control by the public health teams, before it can once again become a major killer in this country. Mrs. Sutcliffe is helping by raising public consciousness and knowledge about this old enemy, while regaling readers with her gentle reminiscences of the Ozarks and prairies of former times.

Alan Chovil, M.D, M.P.H.

Santa Barbara, California
July 1991

Introduction

Summer of 1946, Audubon, Iowa. My father tossed a suitcase into his Jeep for my year-old sister and me, all of five. Before boosting us in, he bent down to the grass by our old brick sidewalk and gently picked up a Daddy-Long-Legs spider.

He held out his hand to Juanita and me and said to the spider, "Which is the way to Mommy?" The spider paused, then slowly lifted up one leg and pointed south. My father nodded. He put the spider carefully back in the grass. We all got in the Jeep and headed south as we had been directed.

Many hours later my sister and I stood on the lawn of the tuberculosis sanatorium at Norton, Kansas, gazing up at a three or four-story building with many windows, the biggest building I had ever seen."See? Mommy's up there. Can you wave to her?" We couldn't see her, but we waved solemnly.

That was my introduction to the world of tuberculosis. Over the years I heard bits and pieces of my mother's story. I did not get seriously interested until my sister found some old negatives our mother had taken in 1930. She printed them in her darkroom, a stunning group of Ozark Gothic faces. Mother wrote down for us her memories of the people in the photos, including Grandma Cherry, of whom we knew nothing.

In 1990, at the age of 82, our mother began to expand this material into a memoir of her life, then she scrapped it and started over, saying that, actually, her life had been a story of tuberculosis, and she might as well tell it the way it really was. I volunteered to edit and ended up helping with the writing as well, because every time I'd ask my mother about some detail, she'd tell me three more stories that she hadn't written down.

In the midst of the writing, we were amazed to see newspaper headlines about a TB epidemic in U.S. cities. Suddenly, this old disease was on the rampage again, and we had a "relevant" book. So we made sure that its contents would be helpful to anyone who seriously wonders what TB is and how not to get it.

Judy Sutcliffe

Pretty Little Stamps

ONE

When I was in the second grade our teacher came to school one day with a few sheets of colorful little stamps. She divided them carefully into blocks of ten and gave a block to each of us. She asked us to sell them for a penny a piece. It was the first time I had seen Christmas Seals. I didn't know what they were, nor did I care. I just wanted to keep those pretty stamps. Happily, my dad gave me a dime for the teacher, and the stamps were mine. It would be many years before I knew the ravages of tuberculosis and the beneficence of the stamps. Yet the disease was already, secretly, in our family.

My father, John William McVicker, was born on George Washington's birthday, February 22, 1866, on a farm near Zanesville, Ohio. I was proud of him. I knew he was someone special for the flags were always flown on his birthday.

When he was a young man, he heard that the government was urging men to go West. He saddled up his horse, whistled for his fox hounds to follow and headed for the Kansas wheat fields. He staked his claim near Lakin, Kansas, in the Great Bend area, and lived in a dugout for several months.

During the wheat harvest he met George Cherry. George invited him to come to Missouri where men were needed to husk corn in Saline County near Marshall. He'd still have time to get back to prove his claim after harvest.

As they rode into Cherry's village, my father saw a young Ozark girl coming down to the spring for a bucket of water. He'd never seen anyone so beautiful. She was Clara Virginia Brown, born at Iberia, Missouri, on June 14, 1882. Her father died before she was born; George Cherry was her stepfather.

1

It was easy to get an introduction. My parents were married on Christmas Day, 1898. She was 16, he was 32. She refused to leave the Ozarks, so he let his claim lapse and used his harvest wages to buy 80 acres of timber near Montier, Missouri, in Shannon County. He cut and cleared small fields for crops, using the logs to build a one-room log cabin. Thus they set up housekeeping. They had eight children: Mary, Edna, Robert, William, Marjorie, John, Charles and Arnold.

By the time I was born on July 14, 1908, they had outgrown two log cabins. I was born in a new, two-story log house. When enough logs were available to saw into lumber, the neighbors came for a housewarming, and a kitchen was built onto the log house.

My mother loved trees and flowers. A row of maples and pines graced our front yard along with a white picket fence. There were rose bushes, lilacs, spirea, passion vines, mock oranges, peonies, flowering locusts and more. She enjoyed gardening, and she always provided houses for birds. Once when I was very small, she was weeding the onions and noticed a snake crawling up the bird house post after baby birds. She was terrified of snakes, yet she dragged the snake down with her hoe, knowing full well it might fall in her face.

My father told me that the best thing that ever happened in his childhood was stepping on a pitchfork. The tines went completely through his foot and kept him on crutches for three years. Since he was not much good for farm work, his father let him go to school. I used to sit on Dad's lap on the kitchen steps of the old log house, facing the barn so he could keep an eye on his livestock. He would read to me from my brother Bill's hand-me-down primer. By the time I started school in the fall, I knew every word.

When my teacher, Ruth Todd, saw that I knew all the flash cards used in the primer class, she wrote a note to my mother asking that I be given a first reader. Mother, who had to pinch pennies, scolded Dad for making it necessary. Why couldn't I wait until Bill was through with his reader? She refused to buy a book for me, and I had to sit with my brother in our one-room school and share his. I learned to read from the front of his book while he studied from the back.

Eventually, I had my very own first reader, and I cherish its memory—the wonderful fragrance of newness. The old primer was musty and mildewed from being left in the haymow and other damp places. The new book had a green cloth binding imprinted with a red rose.

My parents believed in discipline, wanting us to learn right from wrong. Mother used a peach tree switch occasionally to enforce her teachings to respect other people's property. She made sure that each of us had an empty cigar box to keep our treasures in. There were no locks, only our names. And woe be to anyone who trespassed into another's treasures.

Dad used his leather razor strap but not often. Only once can I recall him using it on me. I had worked all morning carrying rocks to outline a floor plan for a dollhouse under the walnut tree in the backyard. My brother Bill wanted me to come play with him, but I was too engrossed. When I finished, I went into the house to get my dolls. When I came back out, all my rocks were scattered helter-skelter. "You old fool!" I yelled at Bill. "You've ruined my dollhouse."

Dad happened to be coming up the road just then and heard me. He went for his razor strap. Before he used it, he reminded me of the Bible verse that said it were better that a millstone be tied around one's neck and he be dumped into the bottom of the sea rather than to call his brother a fool. Dad assured me that I was his baby girl and that he loved me too much for this ever to happen to me. Thus, he must punish me so I would never forget and call anyone a fool again.

I knew that it hurt my dad. And my tender-hearted brother Bill was crying even harder than I was as the razor strap reddened my bare legs.

On summer evenings in a swing made of log chains hung from the limb of a big oak tree in our front yard, Dad would entertain us younger ones while Mother helped Mary and Edna finish up the supper dishes. The songs he sang were ballads, and they were often plaintive and sad, such as "The Poor Little Orphan Boy," which begins

The snowflakes they were falling
And the howling winds did blow
And a poor little boy half frozen
Came to the lady's door.

Tears would glide down our cheeks as he sang the sufferings of the child, concluding with a relatively happy end as the "lady" answers the little boy,

"My only son has fallen,
My only hope is joy:
As long as I live, a shelter will I give
To a poor little orphan boy."

We were not orphans, then. We had enough to eat, and we did not know that we were poor. My parents had convinced us that we were rich in blessings. With enthusiastic voices we sang with our father in the oak tree swing, our mother's voice joining in from the doorway, dishtowel drooping from her arm, "Count Your Many Blessings," and "I am the Child of a King."

I was, in fact, a freshman working my way through college before I learned that I was classed with the poor.

My mother had just died, and the Christmas Seal doctor came with his nurse, Miss Boldt, to check my younger brothers and me to make sure we had not caught tuberculosis from our mother. I knew by now that the sale of those pretty stamps helped fund the National Tuberculosis Association and its work. Miss Boldt saw my flour-sack underwear as I undressed for the examination. She hurried to tell the Methodist women and they, in turn, scurried to collect a box of rayons to give me.

I was horribly embarrassed. I knew that other girls wore rayons. I had seen them as we undressed and showered before swimming classes. But I was proud of my underwear because my bedfast mother had made them for me before she died. She had told me how to remove the colorful printing on the sacks by whitening them in boiling lye water. She had sewn the garments by hand, and I knew that every stitch was done with love, for she had embroidered tiny pink roses at the neckline of the undershirts and finished the hems of the panties with her delicate feather stitches.

My parents had done the best they could for us. Their wisdom and plain common sense made life wonderful in our early years. But they could not control an invisible and mys-

4

terious speck that crept into our home to cause suffering and sorrow, exactly as it had wrecked the lives of generation after generation of human beings since the beginnings of recorded history: the tubercle bacillus, tuberculosis, consumption, the white plague.

We were as ignorant of the workings of this insidious bacterium as Babylonians in the 6th century B.C. To them as to us, it was a mysteriously wasting disease with a cough, and it killed. Mine was the pivotal generation of medical history. My generation went from total ignorance to knowledge of prevention and alleviation and eventually to chemical control.

My children are free of contamination, at least by me. Yet their generation and those following, due to the miraculous near-eradication of tuberculosis in the United States in the first half of the 20th century, are for the most part blithely unaware of this disease, as if it has been banished from the planet.

It has not disappeared. It continues to kill in Third World nations. It enters this country wherever there are poor immigrant populations forced to live in crowded and unsanitary conditions. It is increasing in the general population. Some whose immune systems are weakened by the HIV virus that causes AIDS are also more susceptible to the tuberculosis bacillus. Once detected, the bacillus can be controlled by a severe dosage of anti-tuberculosis drugs, though the drugs can also cause damage in those over 35. There are even new strains of the bacillus that resist control.

The disease can be easily prevented, but people need to know once again how it passes among us.

The methods of transferring AIDS virus from one person to another are well known and widely advertised: unprotected intercourse with an infected person, transference of blood from an infected person. Yet people have panicked over the mortal danger of AIDS and shunned possible carriers as if they might get the disease from merely hugging and kissing or eating from shared dishes.

That fear is aimed at the wrong disease.

It is tuberculosis, a much more ancient disease than AIDS, which can still be given with a kiss.

Some people choose to seek adventure in far away lands. For some, adventure arrives unsought. It unfolds in narrow and quiet circumstances, invisible to the world, mountainous for the one chosen. For me, it began with Grandma Cherry's spoon.

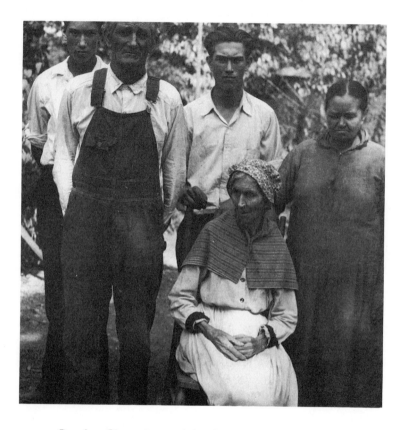

Grandma Cherry is seated. Standing, left to right, are Charles Grover McVicker, John William McVicker, John Joseph McVicker and Minnie Brown. The photo was taken in 1930 in Crocker, Missouri, by Marjorie McVicker.

Grandma Cherry's Spoon

TWO

Grandmother Cherry was not in good health. She had something the doctor diagnosed as catarrh, an inflammation of the mucous membranes of the nose and throat, and she had a stomach ailment. The doctor was a great believer in the medicinal qualities of tobacco. He prescribed a chew of tobacco for the stomach and a corncob pipe for the head.

I remember how my parents described the night my sister Mary climbed on Grandma's lap next to the fireplace. Grandma sat by the fire so she could spit tobacco juice into the ashes. Mary loved her grandmother and liked to mimic her, so when Grandma spat, she would spit, too. Somehow, one of Grandma's tobacco juice missiles landed in Mary's hair. When Grandma saw what a mess she'd made, she gave up the filthy practice that very moment by tossing her corncob pipe and her chewing tobacco into the fire.

When my sister Mary was two years old, Grandma Cherry came to live with our family for a few months to help mother with her first two babies. Edna was a newborn who required much care. So Grandma looked after Mary. At mealtime Mary would sit on Grandma's lap, while Mother held Edna. There were no Gerber baby foods at our table. Mary was fed mashed or cut up foods from Grandma's plate with the same teaspoon with which she fed herself.

Mary grew up tall and sweet. She quit school after World War I when the influenza epidemic hit, and she was needed to help care for sick neighbors. When her boyfriend's little nephews came down with measles, she helped nurse them. Their measles were a different type from the childhood disease that Mary had had, and thus she caught them, too. But she re-

7

fused to give up her plans to be married on Christmas Day, measles or not. She was barely over them when the big day arrived. Dressed in a thin wedding gown, she rode in a buggy to the church. It was a cold, blustery day, and the church was unheated. She caught a cold which reinvigorated the measles and settled in her lungs. She died the next September before her first wedding anniversary and just a week before her 21st birthday. Her illness was called quick consumption.

We were all present at her death, at our home in the room where Mother had cared for her. She did not look ill, just pale and beautiful. First her vision left her, but she asked us all to keep talking to her. Then her hearing began to fade out as well. At the moment of death, she suddenly sat up in bed with a radiant look on her face, calling out, "I see someone coming! Daddy, do you think it could it be Jesus?!"

It was, in fact, acute clinical tuberculosis.

Vigorous little bacillus beasts had gone on a rampage in her body, raging from the walls of the small tubercles her body had built when she was a child to protect her from the primary tuberculosis infection she had sustained from Grandma Cherry. I learned this later from Dr. C. F. Taylor, superintendent of the tuberculosis sanatorium at Norton, Kansas.

He took one look at a photograph of my bony little grandmother, asked if she had ever had close contact with my sister Mary and said that it was highly likely that she had been the source of the family infection.

"She was at a time in life when she had no responsibilities. She was well rested, and the bacilli were held in check," he explained. "She, like many people infected with tuberculosis, had only minor symptoms, yet she may have been a seedbed of the disease all her life."

Mary, like probably everyone in our family, absorbed the initial infection from bacteria that migrated from Grandmother Cherry's spittle. As her sputum dried in the dust, little tuberculosis cells rode away on dust specks in the air, to be breathed in by the unsuspecting. We ran barefoot in the dust. We coughed into cloth handkerchiefs and kept them in our pockets. We knew nothing about germ theory in those days, and we all drank from the same dipper in the water bucket. Mary ate from Grandma's spoon.

No wonder ancient Greek physicians thought tuberculosis was a hereditary, family disease. It was not until 1882 that Robert Koch, in Germany, looked through his microscope at a rod-shaped bacterium which he identified as the cause of tuberculosis.

When tuberculin testing began in schools in the 1920s, it was not uncommon to find 50% or even considerably more of the children showing positive reaction to the test. This response meant that they had been invaded by a primary attack of tuberculosis. Yet they generally appeared in good health. The results of the initial testings were as astonishing to the medical authorities as they were to the childrens' families. The tuberculosis bacillus was everywhere, infecting the general population widely, though only rarely showing external symptoms.

Generally, there were no symptoms of the initial infection that could be detected in children except by the tuberculin test. There were several versions of this revolutionary test. One of the most useful ones, the Mantoux subcutaneous test, was discovered in 1908, the same year that I was born.

The human body's natural defense mechanisms usually worked well, surrounding invading bacteria by walling them off in little tubercles. If the tubercles calcified and were large enough, they could be detected on X-rays. The infected children went on living normal lives and generally showed no further problems. But in the unlucky ones, and luck had about as much to do with it as anything else, the bacteria escaped from the tubercles, often suddenly, with no warning, and could infect any organ or bone of the body.

Why do we rarely see hunchbacks today? Because a major cause was tuberculosis of the spine. The bacillus had a special affection for the lungs, however. The popular form of consumption, romanticized in the tragic stories of Mimi in *La Boheme* and Violetta in *La Traviata*, involved the wasting away of young people in the bloom of life, accompanied by a deadly cough. It was the active reinfection phase after a passive primary childhood infection.

When my sister Mary became bedfast and could no longer take care of her husband and household, the young couple moved in with us. We took care of Mary, washing her dishes with ours. We knew nothing of the possibility of infection at that time. She coughed and spit up stuff, her body quickly consuming itself. When her voice became too weak to call for help, Mother slept with her, because Mary often had smothering spells at night and needed nursing care.

Mother was pregnant with her eighth child at the time. Grieving over Mary's death left her in a weakened condition. Dad took her with John and Charles to Mountain View where they boarded a train for Crocker so Mother could stay with Grandma Cherry and rest up the entire summer.

In the fall, Dad hitched up a pair of mare mules to a two-seated top buggy and took me with him to Crocker to bring Mother and the boys home. It was an adventurous trip for me across the beautiful Ozarks. We slept out at night except for one evening when it rained. A farmer hurried to our camp and insisted we come to the house and sleep on their enclosed porch.

Other than blacksmith shops where we stopped to buy axle grease for our wheels, there were no stores along the way. However, these places were stocked with canned Vienna sausages, crackers and cheese, as well as with gloves and other items travelers might need. Sometimes we stopped at farm houses and tried to buy food. I remember fresh homemade bread with homechurned butter, and tomatoes and onions from the gardens. Yet the people were too generous to accept any money. As we left, I watched Dad throw coins on the grass for the small children. They did not seem to know what money was for.

Dad was protective of Mother on our trip home. At night he wove tree branches together to form a canopy over her head to protect her from the heavy dew. And she enjoyed the food he cooked for us over an open fire. I have no recollection of my grandmother and Aunt Minnie at this, my first visit. My attention was on my mother whom I had missed so much.

Arnold was born in January and was not a strong, healthy baby as all her others had been. We had moved from the two-story log house into our new home built of lumber and closer to the "mail-box" road. Mother's cough continued and she could not regain her strength.

Arnold died of pneumonia shortly after his first birthday.

10

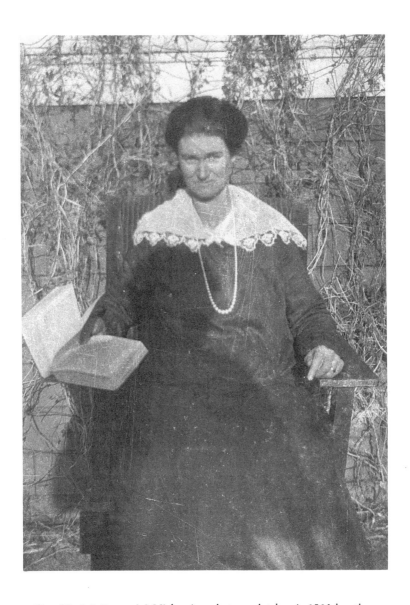

Clara Virginia Brown McVicker, in a photograph taken in 1926, less than one year before her death at the age of 45. She made the chair she sits in.

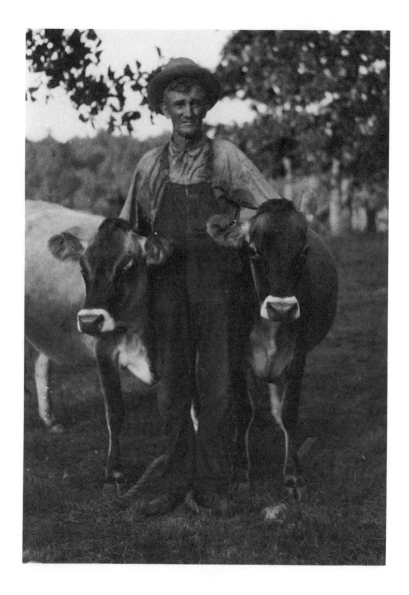

John William McVicker, photographed in 1930 on his farm in
Montier, Missiouri, with his Jersey cows.

Many infant deaths were from acute tuberculosis attacks and Arnold's illness may well have been associated with just such an acute tuberculosis infection. Mother was thrown into a deep depression. She believed that God was punishing her because she was angry when she first learned of this pregnancy, and she had blamed God for letting it happen. There were no birth control pills in those days, and abortions were out of the question. She lost all desire for living. She would go into her room, fondle Arnold's baby clothes and toys and cry for hours. Dad would plead with her to come out and join us at mealtime, to no avail.

By the time she realized that her other children still needed her, she was diagnosed as having advanced tuberculosis. The doctors advised Dad to take her West to a drier climate. Years later, Dr. Taylor told me that if her doctors had said, "go to bed" instead of "go West," my mother might not have died at 45 years of age.

We moved to Elmdale, Kansas, as far West as we could afford. A friend, John Woods, had taken his wife there a couple years previously for the same reason. We were, at least, out of the dampness of the woodlands surrounding our farm.

Dad went ahead of us to find work in the dairy at Clover Cliff Ranch. He wrote home telling us of the fine place we'd have to live in, with lights that needed no match to light them and a bathtub made out of chinaware, just like dishes. Mother was sure he had lost his senses. "How could one get a light without a match just by pulling a string? And such a bathtub! Wouldn't it break from one's weight?"

When we arrived, I was fascinated by an Oliver typewriter in the house of Mrs. Prather, the widow who owned the ranch. She urged me to practice on it so I could help her with her correspondence. It was 1923.

Our apartment turned out to be the maid's or cook's quarters in the large ranch house. My mother's services were required to pay for its use. The widow had five children to cook for in addition to a widowed sister with a teenage son who came for the summer. These and a continual stream of business people and other guests soon became too much for our exhausted mother.

We had expected a miracle from "going West," and didn't

know that the only control for tuberculosis at that time was rest. Mother's instincts were right. She begged Dad to move us into one of the empty tenant houses where she could get some rest. He did, but the first night there, the Cottonwood River went out of its banks, surrounding the house on three sides. Mother slept with one arm reaching down to the floor, feeling for water that might come inside. Luckily, it didn't. Rest was hard to come by.

Little Charles sat by Mother continually, day by day. She'd read the Scriptures to him. If she felt feverish, he'd bathe her face. He ran errands for her.

The Elmdale high school offered cooking classes, and I signed up for them, as I wanted to cook for my invalid mother. The results were not always pleasant. Mother would scream for my brother. "Charles! Charles! I can't eat this awful stuff. Would you cook something for me?" And then she'd tell him how to fix something she wanted. Charles was definitely her favorite, and she occasionally let me know it in no uncertain terms. She was able to sew for me, however, and was happy when she could make me something useful.

The mother of my best friend at Elmdale, Helen Campbell, always welcomed me into their home. She gave me my first permanent waves, and she made my dress for the Junior Prom. Because I was quite tall, dresses from the Sears catalogue did not fit me well. Mother had bought material for a dress for me and was planning to sew it by hand. But the days flew by, and the dance was approaching. Mrs. Campbell suggested I skip school one day and come to her house while she sewed the dress for me, and I decided to let her do it. I didn't realize how much I was hurting my mother. I thought I was saving her trouble because she had no machine and would have had to do it all by hand while lying in bed. It was only later, when I was a mother bedfast with TB myself, that I understood why she shed so many tears over that dress.

She loved to garden, and she couldn't be stopped, sick or not. Somehow she planted her flower bed, using a table fork instead of a hoe. I can remember her crawling back to the house from her garden once, so weak that she could not stand up. She put complete faith in old Dr. Shelley. But we children noticed that every time she told the doctor the medicine he gave her helped, he would always change the prescription.

Mother never let me sleep with her, but I did have a bed in the opposite corner of her bedroom. Shortly after I was graduated from the Elmdale Rural High School in 1927, the County Health officer made his first trip to our home. Mother had been sick for nearly six years and was growing weaker. He brought mother a metal sputum cup and showed me how to unfold a wax paper liner for the cup each morning for her to spit into and how to close up the paper and burn it. He brought a box of paper tissues for her, the first Kleenexes I'd ever seen. Dr. Shelley had never told us of these things.

The County Health officer told me to be sure and boil my mother's dishes. Unfortunately, he did not explain to me that I should boil them BEFORE I washed them. Thinking the heat would make food stick to the plates, I washed them good first and then boiled them. I washed my father's dishes, my two brothers' dishes and my own dishes in the same dishwater as my mother's.

The County Health officer suggested we place Mother in the State Sanatorium for Tuberculosis at Norton, Kansas. He said there were specialists there who might be able to help her.

Later we learned that there were sanatoria in nearly all the states. There was even one in Missouri, and yet my mother's dear, old, trusted Doctor Shelley had never mentioned these facilities to us.

The sanatoria had a twofold purpose, one, to assist tuberculosis patients to regain their health, and, two, to quarantine the infectious tuberculosis carriers from their families and the general population.

The tuberculin tests perfected in the early 1900s were beginning to influence the medical profession and the general public, as more and more was learned about the mysterious workings of the tuberculosis bacillus.

The tuberculin test, originated by Koch and perfected by others, showed who had the bacillus in their bodies and who didn't. Anyone with the primary infection could (though not necessarily would) develop the dangerous and contagious acute reinfection.

The tuberculin tests were simple, safe and accurate. Once they began to be widely administered, particularly in the schools, they revealed where concentrations of infected people were. They prompted health care professionals to start tracking backward through the families to find where the infections were coming from. The tuberculin test helped identify the carriers.

It also influenced the declarations, first by New York's health department, and later by the health departments of most cities and states, that tuberculosis was a communicable and infectious disease and as such reportable in all instances. It influenced the drive to quarantine carriers away from the population at large, in sanatoria.

And so Mother entered the sanatorium at Norton, Kansas, and the rest of us moved to Hays. Hays would put us closer to Norton and allow more visits with Mother. It would also give me the chance to go to college.

The Undertaker's Basket

THREE

Homer Henney, foreman at Clover Cliff Ranch, drove Mother and the rest of our family to the sanatorium at Norton in Mrs. Prather's shiny new Lincoln. We stopped at the sanatorium's greenhouse as we drove in, and Dad bought a dozen carnations. We left Mother in the care of the doctors and nurses there, her thin arms around the bouquet of carnations.

On the way home, we stopped at the Elite Cafe in Hays for lunch. Homer chatted with us and suddenly remembered that there was a college at Hays and an experiment station as well. It was a branch of the agricultural college. He knew Louis Aicher, the superintendent of the experiment station.

Before we left Hays, he had introduced my father to Mr. Aicher, and both my father and my brother John were hired on the spot. John could work part time in the experiment station's nursery, and Dad would have full-time work handling the mules. Mules were used to plow around young trees and in places too difficult for tractors.

I found a part-time typing job in the dean's office, again with good references from Homer. He told them I had worked in his office at the ranch all summer and that my courses in shorthand and typing in high school would enable me to take dictation and help with correspondence.

We found a house to rent within walking distance of the college. Homer used the ranch's big truck to move us to Hays, and on January 17, 1927, I became a freshman in college.

It always seemed to me that I didn't begin to live until I moved to Hays. College classes in psychology, philosophy, public speaking and journalism opened a whole new world to me. Fort Hays (Kansas) State Teachers College was young then, with perhaps 300 students. I recall that the 25th anniversary was celebrated that year with a historical pageant. Everyone seemed open and friendly.

Knowing that I would have to work my way through college, I enrolled in Dr. Gates' business classes. He and his wife had a small son, and I enjoyed invitations to their home.

Once they invited me and other friends to help eat up leftover turkey the day after Thanksgiving. Mrs. Gates asked the women present to accompany her to the kitchen to help put the meal together. When she opened the icebox, we all looked in to find a mangy, sickly kitten nibbling on the turkey we had been planning to eat. Mrs. Gates was very embarrassed, but managed to find something else for supper.

Mr. Gates went in search of their little boy and found him hiding under the bed, way back against the wall. He wouldn't come out, and he wouldn't talk. Later we learned that when he had asked his parents' permission to keep a stray kitten he had found, Dr. Gates had told him to put it in a box. Dr. Gates didn't realize that his two-year-old had only heard of one kind of box in his short life—the icebox.

I enjoyed all of my teachers and classes. In Dr. Start's public-speaking class, I grew in self-confidence. By listening to other students' speeches, I became aware of their feelings and compared them with mine. I also learned how long three minutes can be when one stands before a crowd to speak.

In Lulu McKee's storytelling class, I learned the basics of parenthood and how to help a child develop its mind. Miss McKee told us that all babies love to be held, and if one starts reading to them very early, when still infants, they will associate books with pleasure as well as absorb the rhythm of the language.

Life both in and out of school was full of wonderful new people. Our house on 12th Street had a small chicken house in the backyard. My 14-year-old brother John had insisted on bringing all his pet pigeons and bantam chickens, who took up ready residence. It wasn't long before the lustily crowing roosters brought John a visitor, Edmond Fellers, a boy about his age and similarly equipped with a backyard of bantams, pigeons and fighting cocks just one street away.

I adored my younger brothers and added Edmond to our family flock immediately. His parents, Jay D. and Bessie, had moved to town temporarily to give Bessie a rest, as she, too, was having tuberculosis problems. They owned a farm near Hays.

In the middle of March, the compassionate doctor who was caring for Mother at the sanatorium telephoned for us to come and take her. He explained that she was growing weaker and couldn't live more than a week or two. He felt she would want to spend her last few days with her family.

When we went to fetch her, we found that she had rooted every one of those carnations Dad had given her when she went into the sanatorium.

Mother thought the dismissal meant she would soon be well, and she immediately started to plan a vacation in California. A pen pal had once described to her the giant redwoods and the wild geraniums growing by the roadsides. She had sent photographs, and Mother dreamed of seeing them. She wanted to take her youngest son, Charles, eleven years old, with her.

My sister Edna came from Kansas City with her year-old son, Norman. My brother Bill, not yet married, came from Elmdale. Though we were tearful, Mother was happy to have so many of her children together again. Only Robert, the eldest, was missing. He was married and living on the home place at Montier with his growing family.

Bessie Fellers visited us almost every day with food and comforting words. She seemed to know how much we needed her at that sad time.

Mother died during the night of April 9, 1927. The tubercle bacillus had claimed another victim in our family. It was not yet daylight when Bessie Fellers saw our lights on and guessed what had happened. She and Jay D. hurried to our door.

In the morning, we five children watched the undertaker pick up our mother's fragile, lifeless body and lay it tenderly in his basket. He was carrying her out the door when, through our tears, we saw another neighbor, Wilhelmina Ringe, walking in. She led us to the couch and sat down among us with loving arms around all she could reach. In her German accent she comforted us, "Don't cry now. Your Mutter is gone, but you are mein Kinder now."

It was more than words. She kept us under her wing and never lost touch with us until the time of her death. When I called a few months later to see if I could rent her upstairs room, she said she had just rented it to a construction worker and his wife. "Hold the phone," she said. I heard her endearing accent at the other end of the line calling to the people upstairs, "I vish you move out! Mein girl is coming!"

Dad stayed in Hays, trying to keep our home together. He quit his job at the Fort Hays Experiment Station when he was offered free rent and a higher salary to become the janitor at the Methodist Church. However, he had never worked at an indoor job before, and it was very frustrating, even with help from John and Charles and me.

A girls' dormitory, Wesley Hall, was attached to the church. Frantic girls telephoned day and night to complain that rooms were either too cold or too hot. There was no elevator in the building, and it seemed as if there was always a heavy trunk needing to be moved either upstairs or down.

Then there were the women's organizations with their dinners and activities. Dad continually had to run to the store for another loaf of bread or another pint of cream.

To top it off, the church furnace smoked, and as soon as he would dust off the pews, soot would settle on them again.

Without Mother's help in grooming him, he had trouble looking his best. One morning I came in late to church and saw him sitting alone on a pew up near the front. He looked so lonely and out of place. At first I was embarrassed. His face was smeared with black from the coal furnace. His blue serge suit needed brushing. Then I thought of his love for us in taking this job, and I wanted to be with him. As I walked up the aisle, the congregation stood to sing "What a Friend We Have in Jesus." I touched him on the shoulder and reached for my half of the hymnal.

The church was graced with a hired quartet, directed by the head of the college music department. As if in fear of flatting a note, the voices of the congregation were barely audible. And my dad, who came from country churches where everyone sang for the joy of singing, had also become cautious and conscious of his lack of musical training.

But that morning as I stood close to him, he opened up and

20

sang at the top of his voice. God and His angels must have come to attention! He put so much of himself into each note that he remained one note behind the organ all through the hymn, and I have never known a prouder moment.

Finally, he called it quits. He was homesick for his farm, his friends and his neighbors. He knew he couldn't take us with him, for our sakes. Montier had no high school for John and Charles. And he wanted me to stay in college.

Not long after Mother's death, Jay D. and Bessie Fellers had moved back to their farm. They offered my brother John a home with them. He could stay in school and help Edmond with the chores.

Edna suggested that Charles come live with her family in Kansas City. He could help with her two boys.

I had my job at the college and Dad rented me a room at the Custer Hall dormitory.

Farmers were paying high wages for men to husk corn back in Missouri, so after getting us all settled, he decided to go to work in the cornfields to build up our bank account in Hays. He told me to write checks on the account whenever we needed extra cash. He kissed us all goodby and went home to his farm.

Hays, Kansas, had become special to all of us in a very short time, due to the kindness of friends and neighbors. Charles lasted only one summer in the big city, then ran away, hitchhiking back to Hays. He told me, "Hays is the best town in the world. Hays has the best people in the world, the best schools in the world, and I want to be in Hays."

Charles and I searched for a new place to live. We teamed up with five girls to rent a whole upstairs at Mrs. Mullins' house near the fairground, with three bedrooms for the girls, a cot for Charles in the kitchen plus a bath. Charles found a paper route and on Saturdays was paid to clean out the furnaces for elderly widows. Dividing rent and groceries among seven made it easier for all.

John eventually moved back to town when an apartment became available at the Experiment Station Nursery, where he worked. Even though he no longer lived with the Fellers, they watched over us as if we were their own. Each Christmas Eve they gathered us for an overnight visit to the farm. We opened our packages together by their Christmas tree and ate Christmas dinner with their family. They splurged on gifts for us although we had little but our love to give to them.

Kindness seemed built into the fabric of Hays. Miss McKee and her sister Annie lived near the church and had watched me playing with my little brothers the summer after Mother had died. They knew I loved children, and at an early opportunity, they invited Charles and me into their home. They sat us on a rug beside their shaggy dog, "Tag," and Lulu told us the story of "The Elephant's Child," by Rudyard Kipling. I soon had it memorized myself.

I enjoyed my classes and my teachers at the college. I majored in journalism and English. On the side I took as many storytelling classes from Lulu McKee as I could. Semester after semester swept by, and finally I was a senior.

In the spring of 1930, my doctor thought he saw a weakened spot on my lung X-ray and suggested I take it easy and rest up during the summer. There was still a little money left in Dad's bank account in Hays, so my brothers and I drew it out, spent fifty dollars for a used Model T Ford touring car and drove home to Missouri to spend the summer with our dad.

We cranked up the Model T one day and drove off to Crocker to visit Grandma Cherry. I had seen my grandmother only once before and was eager to get better acquainted.

Halfway there, Dad said, "Turn around, we have to go back. I forgot my teeth." He had always been proud of his mother-in-law and wanted to look his best for her. His "store teeth" were not comfortable, and he only wore them for looks, carrying them in his pocket until needed for show. Luckily, John remembered that Grandmother was blind, so it wouldn't be necessary to go back for the teeth.

I stayed with Grandma Cherry while the others drove in to town. Aunt Minnie had put a chicken in a big pot on the old black range cookstove. As it boiled, the small kitchen sweltered in the heat. Grandma Cherry told me how much she missed doing the cooking and said that Aunt Minnie didn't like to have her in the kitchen. She asked if I would help her gather ingredients, so she could hurry and make dumplings before Minnie got back.

First she asked for a wooden bowl, which she held on her

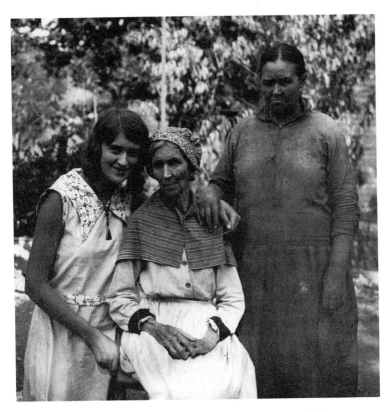

Marjorie McVicker, left, with Grandma Cherry, center, and Aunt Minnie Brown, photographed in 1930.

lap, then for some flour to put in it. She hollowed out a small well with her hand. I wish I could remember what else she asked me to give her to put in it—I only remember her asking me to dip some of the hot chicken broth from the kettle on the stove. She used it as liquid to form the dough, using her fingers. Then she had me roll it out on a cutting board, where she cut it in wide strips lengthwise and then crossways into shorter lengths. Minnie fussed at her when she got back, but I have never tasted better dumplings.

I had a new Kodak box camera, and I photographed my thin little grandmother in her cap and her long cotton dress as she washed dishes in a tin pan on a table on the porch. And Charles snapped her picture with me. It was the last time I saw her. She died of old age within a few years. Many people with tuberculosis have lived to advanced age. The disease's relapsing nature allows periods of inflammation alternating with periods of remission. It does not necessarily kill. In young persons the disease often shows its acute nature, but in old persons, it is more likely to be chronic, with minor symptoms. We did not know at that time that Grandma Cherry had tuberculosis and was infectious. Her cough and her frailty were merely part of old age, it seemed to us, if we even thought about it.

My childhood playmate, Anabelle, came home from Drury College in Springfield that summer. Our fathers had been neighbors and buddies all the years we were growing up. It was a hot, dry summer. With no air conditioning and with no electricity in our homes for fans, we did as many Ozark people do—we spent the warm afternoons swimming. There was a good swimming hole near Camp Witbeck, close to Mountain View, where a crowd gathered each afternoon.

While I was having a good time splashing in the river, the tubercle bacilli were working on the weakened spot in my lung. The doctor hadn't told me that swimming was not the proper way to rest a lung.

Finally, back in Hays that fall, and living at Mrs. Barry's rooming house, I was nearing graduation. I had signed up for fourteen hours my last semester.

One day Mr. Rarick came to me. I had had a teacher's training course with him. He also worked in the college's public relations department.

"You know," he said, "You're going to graduate in January. It's not a good time to start a teaching job. How'd you like to have a job working here for awhile before you start teaching?"

"I'd much rather have a job here!" I answered. "I never wanted to be a teacher in the first place. I just took teachers' training in case I *have* to teach."

"Well," he said, "You're a journalism student, and Mr. Wallerstedt says he needs someone in his printing office here at the college because he can't keep up with all the work. He said he'd like to have you help him because he knows you. He said so at the faculty meeting, and President Lewis said the college would pay you eighty dollars a month and Mr. Waller-stedt would teach you to run the Linotype."

I was excited at this news. I had been skipping meals and working during my noon hours as well as after classes in order to get in as many hours of work as I could. I kept a box of raisins in my desk drawer, so if my stomach started to complain at noon, I'd just eat a few raisins. But even with the extra noon hours, at thirty cents an hour I couldn't make more than thirty-five dollars a month. That had to pay the room rent for Charles and me, plus our food and my college expenses.

So I thought to myself, "Well, gee, with eighty dollars a month I could get John back in high school." He hadn't been out long.

I accepted the offer from the college immediately. I agreed to start Linotype lessons with Mr. Wallerstedt the very next morning.

That happy evening, when I went to supper at the rooming house, Mrs. Barry served us a cabbage salad with peanuts in it. There were about twenty of us at the table. We were laughing and acting foolish, as usual. I choked on the salad. I excused myself and ran upstairs to the bathroom.

Every time I'd cough, I'd spit in the stool. And every time I spat, it was blood, a bloody foam. Finally, I called Mother Barry upstairs to tell her something was wrong. I didn't know what the matter was, but I was bleeding.

The People in Hays

FOUR

"Well,'" Mrs. Barry said, "Something's wrong. I'm going to call the doctor."

"I guess I can do that myself," I said. I reached for the nearest phone and called Dr. Morris from the college. He lived just a few houses away.

He said, "You get to bed. And don't put a pillow under your head. Get as flat as you can, and I'll be right over."

In a few minutes he ran up the stairs. He said to me, "Oh, honey, you're having a hemorrhage. You've got to go to bed and stay there."

I had heard of tubercular chest hemorrhages, for my mother had greatly feared having one, yet she suffered for six years without one occurring. My sister also did not hemorrhage.

With the flow of blood from my lungs, my life was changed. I never went back to school. I did not finish my degree. I did not learn the Linotype. I lay quiet and still in that bed at Mrs. Barry's and waited to see what would happen.

Hemorrhages were rather rare. A tubercular lesion that opened into a large blood vessel could cause a hemorrhaging person to pour forth blood from the lungs and to bleed to death. I was lucky. In my case, the hemorrhaging blood vessel was a small one. The hemorrhage was, in fact, something of a "smoke detector" that showed my doctors a serious problem was imminent, in time to do something about it.

The next day the Methodist preacher announced in church that I had had a hemorrhage. Bouquets started to arrive from the sororities and fraternities. My little bedroom was full of flowers and kids.

A boy I'd been dating heard that I was sick. When he came to see me, he found me laughing with my friends and surrounded with pretty flowers. He said, "Well. I thought you were supposed to be sick, but I think you feel better than I do, and I quit work early to come see you, too." He was angry with me and never came to visit me again.

In the next day or so the nurse from the college came. She said, "I've got good news to tell you, Marjorie. President Lewis mentioned at the faculty meeting that you were sick, and people began to hand out money. They just emptied their billfolds. And so we're going to take you to the Protestant Hospital."

"If I have TB," I replied, "then I don't mind going to the sanatorium where my mother was."

But the nurse continued. "You know, it didn't take very long at all, and we had over seven hundred dollars. That will pay your hospital bill for a good while. We don't think you look that sick, and if you're put in a sanatorium with advanced cases, you might get more infection. We're going to take you to the hospital here, and Dr. Morris will take care of you."

The nurse told me she had a list of names of the people and the amounts they had given. I told her not to show me the list. I did not want to value my friends by the amount of money they could give. So she told me of only one—a new professor who said he had forgotten to give me a test paper to mimeograph until the end of the day, and that I had stayed overtime to do it, then delivered it with a smile.

That was October 1930. Dr. Morris placed me in Hays Protestant Hospital. He came to see me every day. He never missed.

Others came, too. One day a stylishly dressed old gentleman walked into my room and inquired, "Who in hell are you, and what are you doing in this hospital?"

I explained that I had hemorrhaged, and the doctor had put me here to rest. He introduced himself as Alex Phillips and continued, "I was a young man working in a bank in London when I first spat up blood. I kept on working, and when it got to the place I was spitting up more blood than they liked, I left the bank job and came to America.

"I came out here to western Kansas, where I could spit up all the blood I damned well pleased. I got me a horse, a kettle

27

and a blanket and a job on the range. I rode the range all day, slept with my blanket on the good earth at night and cooked my beans over an open fire in the kettle. And I am as healthy as a gopher.

"Let me tell you, young lady. You get out of this bed and go out to my ranch. They will saddle you up a horse, and you can ride in fresh air all day and eat all the good food you want at my son Bill's table. It is still my ranch, and I am the boss, but he runs it, and he's a god-damned good manager."

I soon learned that this astonishing man and his wife had spent some time in the same hospital, so now it was his hobby to walk the halls every day and make the rounds of the patients, whether he knew them or not. He became a dear friend to me. Once the Presbyterian minister to whose church the Phillips belonged asked me if Alex swore when he talked to me. I told him, no, he just talked in his natural way, which I didn't consider swearing at all as there was no anger or bitterness in his tender and understanding heart.

One day his wife phoned to tell me he was bringing me a bowl of hot soup and to watch for him through the window. She often brought home the bones of the turkey carcass after a church turkey dinner. She simmered them for broth and made a delicious barley soup.

Alex arrived at my door, but close behind him came his wife. I was delighted to see her as she explained, "Alex, the old rascal, I was afraid he would stop to talk and let it get cold."

Thoughtfulness from people who hardly knew me was a common occurrence. I recall one day when Mr. Moody, the beloved old popcorn man on Hays' Main Street, stopped a first grader after school and asked if he would take a sack of free popcorn for himself and another for Marjorie who was in the hospital. The little boy happened to know me, as he was Bessie Feller's nephew. He gladly set off to make the delivery, but when he reached the hospital, a nurse told him that children were not allowed to visit the patients.

Lloyd waited until the nurse left, then he slipped up the stairs, found my room and delivered the popcorn. When he heard footsteps he quickly hid behind my door. When it was safe to come out, his shirt caught on my thermometer, and it fell to the floor. He saw the shattered glass and tried to pick it up.

Then he looked up at me and said, "The silly thing should never have been made of glass no how."

And then one day, it was spring, and Dr. Morris told me my X-rays showed I had improved a bit. I could get up, and he'd try to find a rooming house for me so I could leave the hospital. He said I could work about an hour a day, if I took it easy.

I told him, "When you go to those rooming houses, you be sure and tell them that I have TB, because I'd hate to move in to somebody's house and then have them find it out."

He came back that evening and said, "Margie, I can't get you a room if I tell them you have TB. Right away they say, no, they won't take you. I've got to get you a room, and I —I just have to not tell them."

"Well, it's going to be terrible if I get in a room and then they find it out. I'd feel awful." He went away, and I settled down and prayed.

In the next day or so, in came Nellie Sites. She was a little girl with a humpback, but she had always been my friend. Her parents said she'd been dropped down the stairs when she was little, but I often wondered if she had not had tuberculosis of the spine, though her parents may not have known it. She came in the room and said, "Margie, we heard they were going to move you out of the hospital and that you needed a rooming house. My mother sent me up here to tell you to come to our house. We'd love to have you."

I said, "Well, Nellie, I have tuberculosis. You might get it."

"No," she said, "Mother said we had a room for you all by yourself, and there'd be no danger. You come and stay with us."

Dr. Morris gave me instructions before I moved into Sites' house. "You stay in your room as much as you can. We'll get you a meal card, and you can walk up the street to the restaurant to eat. It's best if you don't go into the family quarters at all, unless they ask you to. It's better not to mingle with the family."

The only way to the front door was through the living room. The old man and his wife were always sitting there when I walked through. One evening when I came back, Mrs. Sites said, "Well! We always thought you were a real friend of ours. But we didn't know you were so snooty that you wouldn't associate with us after you got here. All you do is stay in your room. You don't come out. That's not the way to live in the family."

After that, one of their sons, John Sites, who had returned to Hays after attending the University of Chicago, came to my room every day to just sit and talk with me.

Dr. Morris said, "If they want you to mingle with them, well, mingle with them." So I would stop in the living room and visit with them before I walked to the restaurant.

Then one day Mrs. Sites said to me, "Margie, you know you're paying money uptown eating out every day. We have food here, and there's no reason on earth you couldn't eat with us. We could sure use the money."

So Dr. Morris said, "Okay, if they want to do it that way, we'll pay them for the food instead of the restaurant." So I ate at Mrs. Sites' house. She was certainly a good cook, much better than the restaurant, and I was considered non-infectious now, since the hospital couldn't find any sign of TB bacillus in me.

I had started to work for Dr. Rarick in the public relations office an hour or so a day. One afternoon there was a lovely light drifting of snow on the sidewalks. Dr. Rarick looked at me and said, "How come you aren't wearing overshoes?"

"It's all right," I said. "I don't have any, and it's not snowing very much."

That night when it was time to go home, Dr. Rarick came to me with a pair of brand new overshoes. He'd gone uptown and bought me a pair. He made me put them on, and then he drove me home in his car.

Most people were afraid of catching TB from someone who had shown symptoms, so I stayed to myself much of the time. When Dr. Rarick invited me to his home for dinner one Sunday, I politely refused, thinking his wife might not really want me around her family. The next Sunday as I was leaving the church, Mrs. Rarick invited me to dinner, but I again refused. A few moments later, her son Lawrence stepped up to invite me. I still refused. Daughters Margaret and Lois ran to ask me next. Dr. Rarick caught me at the door, "Do you feel like you've been invited enough? If so, let's go to the car. I'm getting hungry!"

30

That was the way people treated me in Hays.

I had barely been working for him for two weeks, when in the middle of the night I began to cough, and I could taste blood. It was the bloody foam again. I thought of all the people who had been paying for my hospital bill, the rooming house, and now I was bleeding again.

I really believe that at that moment if I'd had poison I would have taken it, because I didn't want anybody to have to take care of me.

But there I was with nothing but a box of Kleenexes, all of them full of blood. When John Sites came in to see me the next morning, he saw all this blood and called the doctor right away.

They moved me back to the hospital immediately. John Sites came over to the hospital room that morning with a recipe card that he wanted me to keep with me, no matter what happened. He had written a verse on the back of it.

The world is filled so full of joy
That little woes can ne'er destroy—
What if some sorrow does come my way,
I'll smile at it and simply say:
"Of one fair blessing I'm bereft,
But, oh, I have a million left."

It reminded me of the old gospel songs my parents taught us to sing at our family altar after breakfast. Mother would pick up Dad's plate and replace it with the Bible. He would read from it, and then all seven of us would kneel beside our chairs for prayers. My knees often hurt and the prayers seemed long, but I always looked forward to the gospel hymns afterwards. My parents loved to sing, and I remember them singing, "God Will Take Care of You."

Sleeping on the Porches

FIVE

This time I insisted that I be taken to the state sanatorium. No longer could I allow my friends to pay my hospital bills. It was up to me to take charge of my life and do the best possible. But I was feeling terrible to think that the county would have to pay my bill at the sanatorium.

In the midst of my depression, Dr. Morris told me to quit feeling bad about the money. He said, "You know, your dad has paid taxes all these years, and the reason he has paid taxes is for these sort of things to be available if you need them. So don't worry about your being on the county, you're entitled to it." I wonder if welfare patients are treated so nobly today.

In July 1931, Tony Gross, the college driver, and a nurse took me to Norton. I knew Tony because he had driven for two trips to Estes Park, Colorado, when I was a delegate to the annual YWCA-YMCA conferences there.

When Tony asked if I liked strawberry ice cream sodas and learned I had never had one, he insisted on stopping in Norton to treat me to one before driving on to the sanatorium, which was five miles outside of town. When he drove away, I was left among strangers.

There were normally about 150–200 public patients at the sanatorium and a few private patients. In addition to three doctors, which included the superintendent, Dr. C. F. Taylor, the staff of nearly 150 included nurses, lab technicians, administration, cooks, yardmen and farm employees. Much care was needed to nurse the patients back to a state of health.

Dairy products were an important part of every meal for patients, to supply needed calcium. Thus a dairy farm was an important part of the complex. Even the ancient physicians of Greece had prescribed milk and eggs for tuberculosis sufferers, perhaps because their patients so often appeared emaciated.

Hippocrates, who was born in 460 B.C., termed the wasting illness *pthisis,* meaning both to melt and to waste away. He treated the disease by assisting nature's natural healing capacities through providing adequate diet, good nutrition and control of symptoms with a minimum of drugs, very much the same techniques used by the sanatoria of the 1930s.

The Norton sanatorium included one main hospital building, eight residential pavilions with screened-in porches, a dining hall, nurses' home, superintendent's residence, post office, greenhouse and an employees' building. A small creek ran through the grounds, which covered a considerable acreage and included cropland for the cows.

One of the eight pavilions was a private WOW (Woodmen of the World) Insurance building, financed and built by the insurance company, but staffed by the state. I didn't have any insurance, nor did most of the other public patients. But Dr. Taylor wouldn't leave any bed empty in that more handsomely appointed two-story, brick building, which had room for 12 women and 12 men. If there was a bed free, county patients would be put there, as I was, initially, though I was later moved to the public buildings.

Twenty patients were housed in each of these long, usually one-story, wood-frame pavilions with screened porches along one side. There were ten patients lined up in beds in each screened wing, with a reception room for visitors and a kitchen area separating the two sections. Nurses lived on the other side of the building, at least two nurses per pavilion. I was in the newest of the public pavilions, Pavilion Seven, which was a two-story brick building with a capacity of forty. Men and women were in separate pavilions, and in the 1930s, blacks were segregated from whites, though Dr. Taylor changed that by the mid 1940s. Children also had their own pavilion.

Food was cooked in a central dining hall and distributed to the pavilions in heated carts. Nurses then took food trays to each bed. Dr. Taylor monitored the nurses carefully to be sure that all the patients were receiving warm meals.

The patients spent most of their time in bed on the screened porches. This included sleeping on the porches in the open air at night. Fresh air was thought to have an invigorating effect on the body, and patients were thoroughly supplied with fresh Kansas air, winter and summer.

There were canvas blinds at each bed with ropes to unwind in case of a storm. Many times I awoke to find my bedcovers white with snow, because I failed to awaken and let the blinds down.

In winter we were told to wear extra pairs of cotton flannel pajamas for sleeping plus a double-thickness, flannel night cap with strings that tied under our chins. Each bed, happily, was equipped with an electric heating pad which made these fresh air bedrooms bearable. There was a small private room at the end of each bed, just large enough for a dresser and for the wheeled bed itself, when it was pulled in for the patient's morning bed bath twice a week. The screened-porch area was open, so that the nurses could walk up and down the porch from bed to bed.

In later years, the fresh air treatment lessened in importance as doctors discovered that it was rest and diet alone that seemed to be controlling the disease. But air in some form had been a preoccupation of health care providers since the early Greek physicians: fresh air, high altitude air as in Thomas Mann's *Magic Mountain*, air from volcanoes, dry air, hot air, cold air, even lack of air, all were prescribed at one time or another for tuberculosis patients throughout history.

As soon as I was assigned a bed and had gotten myself organized, I wrote to my sister Edna in Kansas City that I had hemorrhaged again and was in the sanatorium. She wrote back to tell me that she had spit up blood plenty of times herself, but she never went to bed, she just kept on working. She was disgusted with me for what seemed to her the lazy way of dealing with tuberculosis. She did not communicate with me the rest of the time that I was at Norton.

I was pretty miserable the first few weeks. One day I was writing a letter to my father who was living alone on the home place in Missouri. I wondered how I could find a special way to let him know how much I cared about him and loved him.

Once in a college literature class, Dr. Macgregor had told us about parodies and assigned us to write one. I struggled all evening and finally gave up and went to bed. During the night I woke up with a start, saying to myself, "Dr. Macgregor will get you if you don't watch out!"

I realized immediately that it was a parody of the "Little Orphan Annie" poem I had read many times. I hurried to put it on paper. Words came easily and rhymed. Dr. Macgregor was so pleased with it next morning that he read it aloud to the class, laughing so hard he could barely say the words.

Remembering the fun I'd had with that poem, I began to practice making up poems as I lay in bed. Soon I was writing rhymed verses about my childhood and my dad and enclosing them with my letters to him. He loved them and began clipping Edgar Guest poems from his newspaper to send to me.

Verse writing became a hobby. I used my poems to express my appreciation to all the people who were good to me. I had never met the cook at the hospital, but I enjoyed the food, so I wrote a verse to thank her and left it on my tray. She was surprised and delighted to find it and hurried up the elevator to bring me her thanks. I wrote verses to the janitor and to the little German-Russion girl who came each morning to wake me and clean my room. Another poem was for the nurse who gave me wonderful alcohol backrubs each evening before bedtime.

I learned how important it is to develop a hobby one can pursue if forced to be confined to bed for any length of time.

I don't know what I would have done during those long days and months in the sanatorium if I had not enjoyed reading books. Most of the patients on our porches liked to read, but once in a while we'd get one who did not read or have a hobby, and she would provide enough misery to depress all of us. One by one the others would get up and pull their beds into their rooms to escape her. Not wanting to be rude, I often remained the only one on the porch listening to her grumble. I vowed then if I ever had children, I would encourage them to read and to develop hobbies.

I spent three years at the sanatorium in Norton. After the first few months I stopped asking when I could go home. They'd say, "Well, you're a lot better, but it will be, maybe, another month or so." They'd never say it would be two or three years.

But everyone was kind. And I had visitors. The first person who came to see me was John Sites. He wanted to take me with him out West. He'd take care of me, he said. "No, I'm going to stay right here," I replied. "This is where I need to be."

One of my next visitors was an old man from Norton, Oscar Miller, who walked the five miles from his home to the sanatorium carrying a limb from his cherry tree. He walked up and down the pavilions, letting us all pick cherries. He came often to see us, always bringing something from his garden.

President Lewis from the college came to see me. And the Presbyterian preacher, Reverend McCleave. He always said we were kin, because he was crippled and walked with a cane. Tuberculosis had affected his bones when he was a child.

Dr. Taylor even brought the governor of Kansas and his legislative delegation around to look at us all, from a safe distance. We felt just a little as if we were in a zoo. One of my porchmates quipped as the governor left, "Peanuts, anyone?"

Dr. Taylor lived in a spacious home near the entrance of the sanatorium and not far from the pavilions. He was a man of medium height with a stocky build and round face. He had a resonant baritone. One morning early he went out on his porch and sang, "Ah, Sweet Mystery of Life." His voice wafted clear and strong to all our beds. He and his wife had two daughters and four sons, several of whom grew up to be doctors. The children were not allowed to enter any of the pavilions, but they were great entertainers as they visited us from outside the screened porches. One boy brought large bull snakes and let them coil about his shirtless body as we watched and shrieked.

Dr. Taylor's clan included a set of twins, and one of them, Danny, seemed to always be in trouble. When Danny started stealing art materials at school, though he had plenty of his own, Dr. Taylor surmised that he was not getting enough attention at home. He bought him a fishing pole and spent many hours fishing with him. That helped matters considerably. But as time went on, more problems arose. One evening we heard Dr. Taylor's beautiful voice singing from his porch with deep feeling, "Danny Boy." In his first year of college Danny died in a car wreck.

Dr. Taylor spent a lot of time with me and patiently explained the hows and whys of tuberculosis, as well as he and other health professionals understood it at that time. I began to understand the way in which it had spread throughout my family, and I determined that it would go no further.

Dr. Taylor liked to talk to me, and would often call me to his office, which had the hide of a big old Holstein bull on the floor. My porchmates were a little jealous. They called me "Taylor's Pet" and would ask, "How come you always get to go sit on the bull and not us?" Sometimes he'd take me for a drive in the country. He would talk and talk about the things that were bothering him. He had come from a poor family in Chicago and had vowed to make something of himself. I was a sounding board for him as he worked out the problems of the sanatorium and his life. So was "Torgy," the lab technician, Miss Torgeson. Both of us were friends with whom he could freely talk, because he could trust our confidence.

Dr. Taylor had more influence on my life than anyone outside of my parents. He admired me because I had gone to college, while working to support myself. There were few patients at the san who had attended college. He wanted me to write and asked me to help him in many of his writing projects.

He was always up to something new. Once he trapped so many beavers in the creek that he was able to have a fur coat made for his wife. He was very proud of that. He was a good photographer, and the hospital walls were lined with framed black and white photographs of landscapes that he had taken. He also wrote poetry. But it was blank verse, unlike my own, and I couldn't quite understand it.

He pondered questions about TB that didn't have answers. One day he said, "You know, I'm not a church fan, but I'm going to build an all-faith chapel. I've noticed that a lot of people with a strong faith in God have something extra to carry them through. They survive." He was disgusted with the rantings and wranglings of the various denominations and determined to build something non-denominational. It would be constructed of beautiful wood. In a few years this was accomplished.

One of our ministering angels was a public health nurse, Miss Maude Boldt. It was she who had first come to our home in Hays after my mother's death had been reported to the National Tuberculosis Association. It was she who had supplied me with my first rayon lingerie and with two dresses from her closet. When I arrived at the "san," as we called it, there she was, too, employed as a personal relations nurse serving all the patients. She was a woman of indefatigable energy. She visited the sick hour after hour, cheerfully raising their spirits and invigorating them with her own strength. She would go to town to do our shopping for us. By the time I was given permission to exercise, she had started a library, and I helped carry books to those who were not yet allowed to walk. She was the personal confidant for many people confined to their beds. She listened to them, responding to their emotional needs. Her life was consumed in helping others.

When old age finally caught up with her, and the doctor said she was no longer capable of living alone, she found it hard to adjust. She who had always cared for others could not accept helplessness for herself nor the offer of care from the administration of the sanatorium. But she dressed for the occasion. When they found her lifeless body down by the creek, she was wearing her black corset and her very best black lace underwear.

I thought of her whenever I loaded a cart with books to take to patients who were not able to come to the library. The sickest cases were in the hospital building on what we called, "death row."

Dr. Taylor told me to sit down and listen if any of them were anxious to talk. He was certain they'd speak to another patient more freely than to a doctor. He felt it was good therapy for them to talk but urged me to respect their confidences.

My chest hemorrhages had never caused me any pain or suffering, but here were people who suffered constantly.

One was an eleven-year-old Mexican lad whose father had died. He talked of getting well fast, so he could go home to help support his mother and younger brothers and sisters. Tuberculosis had spread all through the child, even to his stomach. He had trouble eating, because he couldn't digest his food. He begged the authorities to give him the Mexican food he was used to and loved, but when he explained what he wanted, the doctors shook their heads and said his frail little body couldn't survive it. He died soon after.

Death from tuberculosis seems to have plagued mankind since shortly after Eden. It was a known killer in India and China two and three thousand years B.C. In more recent centuries, in London the death rates ranged from 20% in 1667 to nearly 33% dying from TB in 1799. When records were first kept in Massachusetts in 1842, 22% of all deaths were recorded as due to tuberculosis. Deaths began to drop in the United States from about that time on, due to better environmental conditions, and, later in the century, the growing prevalence of sanatoria which isolated carriers from the rest of the population. Seven states had sanatoria by 1907, and by 1942, there was a state sanatorium in each of 42 states, as well as a considerable number of private institutions. The United States death rate from tuberculosis at the turn of the century was nearly 200 per 100,000 population. By 1930, this was down to only 75, and by 1950, around the time that anti-tuberculosis drugs became available, the death rate had already sunk to only 25 per 100,000.

This great drop in the tuberculosis death rate was due to sanatoria quarantine of carriers, to near-eradication of the disease in cattle, along with early diagnosis through the tuberculin test and prevention of the disease through health education campaigns of the National Tuberculosis Association. Still, superstition and lack of scientific knowledge prevented compassionate understanding in a few.

Local ministers took turns preaching sermons to us from a safe distance over a loud speaker system that went to each bed through a set of earphones. One minister evidently thought it would be to his glory if he could save the souls of all of us who were sick. As I listened to his hell and brimstone message, I thought of the brave children on "death row." It bothered me so much I wrote the minister my objections.

The next morning I found one boy very disturbed. He asked me if I had heard the sermon. I sat down and took his warm little hand in mine. I assured him that the minister was wrong, that God loved him and that Jesus had come to tell us that God was like a loving father, and we need not ever be afraid. He died the next day.

I was ashamed of some of those ministers. They wanted the glory of saving our souls, but not if we or our families weren't giving a little money to the church. They were great at lecturing on sin, but they were not much good at sitting with the sick and just visiting.

Other ministers were more understanding. Father Mulvahill was the Catholic priest in Norton. He made frequent visits to the san and regaled us with rollicking stories of his boyhood in Ireland.

Reverend DeYoung, a Dutch Reform minister from a neighboring town, rallied his congregation to pack picnic lunches once a week and form a caravan to come visit the people at the sanatorium. They would spend the entire day visiting patients, and in the evening he would deliver a loving and caring message to all the patients by radio.

The radio was one of our delights. When we took my mother to the sanatorium in 1927, we promised to buy her a crystal set like the ones several of our neighbors had acquired. After she'd been there a short time she wrote us not to get her a radio. She said she preferred a phonograph because she could shut it off.

When I entered the san in 1931, radios were more common, and a few patients had them. Soon those who did were forced to wear earphones in order not to disturb other patients. But many of the patients yearned to hear the programs. The solution came in the person of a former patient named Danny. He had taken a correspondence course in radio and was now employed as an electrician at the san. He volunteered to run wires to every pavilion with plug-ins at every bed so each patient could tune in to a central radio station run by the men's pavilion.

We greatly enjoyed Amos & Andy, Bing Crosby, Don Ameche and other radio personalities of the day. Statewide news releases from the sanatorium let the public know that the sanatorium needed earphone sets. People all over Kansas mailed us the headphones from their outdated crystal sets. Al and Jane Esterdahl of Hays sent me theirs. I wrote to thank them, and we struck up a correspondence that lasted for years.

Dr. Taylor now used the radio instead of the little newspaper he had tried hard to establish for his news and announcements. He thought my journalism experience would make it grow, but my work was of little use. The news from the staff was too dull. We couldn't compete with Charlie Grubbs' carbon-copied "Sanatorium Scandals." Charlie had fought TB most of his life. He had sowed wild oats all over the world, and he had the gift of gab. He successfully peddled his papers for a dime apiece, whereas the free sheets from the doctors were seldom read.

Charlie always had a ready source of news from life on the porches.

The People of the San

SIX

Tubercle bacilli do not discriminate. They attack all classes of people. My porchmates were rich, poor, Protestant, Catholic, educated and uneducated, black and white. And mostly young. Often tuberculosis was the only thing we had in common. We were all different, and I soon learned not to expect the others to think like me.

A divorced woman patient was nicknamed "Sinner" by a few patients who didn't approve of her lively sexuality. There was a strict rule against patients dating each other. She was caught several times sneaking out at night with one of the men patients. One or two men had been expelled from the san because of her, but she couldn't be expelled because she was a member of the WOW Lodge and was not under the supervision of the state authorities.

She had a great sense of humor which brightened our days, and she was always the first to greet new patients and help them adjust to the routine of sanatorium living. She told me bits and pieces of her life story. She had married young, and, after a third baby's arrival, she realized that marriage was not all fun and romance. The responsibilities and hard work mounted. She and her husband divorced. She soon decided she'd made a mistake, but when she looked up her ex-husband, she found he'd already married again. After that she broke down with tuberculosis and had to give up custody of the children. It seemed to her as if the world were against her, and so she lived from day to day, taking pleasure where she could and not worrying about the consequences of broken homes and other people's misery. She warned me if I ever married to think twice before asking for a divorce because most reasons later seemed far too small.

Some romances fared better. One of my good friends at the sanatorium was Etna. When she entered the san, her lungs were ravaged "like a sieve," according to Dr. Taylor. But she had a strong will to live and a vibrant personality, and she survived. She met Pete, who was Swedish, at the sanatorium, and they married while still within its gates. After leaving the sanatorium, they had one child, a boy, and bought a motel. Dr. Taylor puzzled over the difference between Etna and her sister, who also was a patient. The sister was far less seriously affected with TB than Etna, but she had children at home and worried herself sick. She died in a very short time.

The desperation of a few patients drove them into the hands of quacks. A young woman on my porch told me in broken English that her father brought her family to the United States from Germany shortly after World War I. She had been in love with a young man in their home town, but her father forbad their marriage. She resorted to pregnancy as a convincing argument and thus brought Richard with her to the U.S. as her husband. She fell ill with advanced TB while caring for their baby. I asked if I might read to her, as she was very ill, but all that she had was a German Bible. I found in the library information on the phonetic pronunciation of the German language, and so I read to her in German, though I had no idea what I was saying. Her husband, fearful for her life, felt that she was not making enough progress at the sanatorium. He came to take her away one day, saying that they would go to a man in South Dakota who effected miracle cures by manipulating the body. I never found out whether she survived. Dr. Taylor feared that if the quack doctor put pressure on her chest and lungs, she could easily hemorrhage.

Most of my porchmates were adult young women, but occasionally a child was placed with us. Emily was a very young girl with such an advanced case of tuberculosis the staff did not want to put her in the children's pavilion. We were delighted to have her on our porch, but were surprised when she asked for dirt to eat. She was from a southern state, and the doctors explained to us that she had been raised in an area where most diets were very poor. People there seemed to recognize that they were deficient in minerals and attempted to add them to their diets by eating dirt. Emily was not supplied with any western Kansas dirt on her dinner trays, however. One day she saw an ad in the local paper for a special kind of candy and begged a nurse to buy her some. But Emily was disappointed when she tasted it, "Ummph! Just plain old lickrich!" She had seen the word "licorice" in the ad but had pronounced it to herself as "lice-a-rice."

It was fun to have a child in our group, since at that time I was still confined to bed and could not visit other areas.

I recall a nurse's story of an incident in the children's pavilion involving a little eight-year-old boy. When she made her rounds to see that each child was tucked in for the afternoon rest period, Jimmie was missing. She called another nurse, and they searched the premises to no avail. Since Jimmie was a sweet and obedient little boy, they decided his mother must have come to take him for a ride in the country. She was a widow employed by one of the diet kitchens.

When Jimmie didn't show up after rest hour, they phoned the mother, but she hadn't seen him since noon. Superintendent Taylor was notified, and a thorough check of the grounds and the sanatorium farm was made. The farm was a temptation to boys who wished to play hookey from bed. News traveled quickly along the grapevine from one sleeping porch to another, and speculation mounted as to what might have happened to Jimmie—hot summer day...nearby creek...poor Jimmie.

A nurse found him when she went to get a sheet from the linen closet. He was sound asleep on the very top shelf. Yes, he had a reason. He was playing Pullman and took his afternoon rest period on the top berth.

Jack Cunningham, a former patient who stayed on to become the sanatorium postmaster, was the highlight of our days when he made the rounds with the mail. Jack knew of my interest in children and often told me what went on in the children's pavilion.

Once he related that every morning when he opened the door, he would see a long hall with twenty doorknobs and a pajama-clad youngster clinging to each. Always he heard the same mixed chorus:

"Any mail for me, Jack? Any mail for me?"

"Darn," he said. "It began to get to me. Some of these little tykes never received any letters or packages. But every morning there they were, just as hopeful as those who did.

"Then I hit on the idea of sending them the second and third class mail which I'd been tossing in the waste basket. I readdressed circulars and catalogues to Betty and Billy and Joan and Jack. For a morning or two, I hung around just to see how those little devils' eyes would light up when the nurse called their names.

"A week or two later, the teacher from the sanatorium school asked me about Betty. It seemed this eight-year-old who had been a good student suddenly took a drop for the worse. Her teacher kept her in for questioning one day.

"'You know, Miss Allen,' explained Betty, 'I have been getting so much mail here lately, I just haven't had time to look at my books.'

"Doggone!" concluded Jack, "it sounds silly, but I don't know when I ever got a bigger kick out of anything."

Although most of the older patients at the sanatorium had tuberculosis of the lungs, the children were afflicted with a greater variety of tubercular possibilities. Sometimes bones were infected, sometimes glands and membranes. There were two little boys I knew whose bones were diseased, though I couldn't detect this by looking at them, as they were not advanced cases. Dr. Taylor asked me if I'd entertain them, and we'd meet outside on the lawns and tell stories together. One had parents who came to see him, and the other had a mother who visited. For some reason they were not pavilioned with the other children; perhaps they were among the WOW insured patients.

Once I was on my feet again, I began to meet more patients. There was an old man in the WOW Lodge building who had worked in lead mines. His lungs were full of lead, and he talked in barely a whisper. He was a devil of a fellow, always teasing the women. Without thinking about it, women tended to respond to his sallies in whispers as soft as his.

I especially liked Johnnie, a Croatian from Kansas City. He was married to a Croatian woman, and their first baby was born while he was in the sanatorium. But she divorced him before he was able to leave. TB was hard on marriages.

Wally, the elderly janitor, in his younger days also had been a patient. Tuberculosis had cheated him out of the opportunity to marry and build a home of his own, so he'd stayed on at the san. He never lacked for love, however, for every girl in the place was in love with Wally. It was Wally who ran the Wheelchair Bus Line. Whenever a patient who wasn't allowed to walk needed to go to the hospital for treatment, X-rays, or lab tests, it was Wally who was sent for. His gentle, cheerful nature made these trips with Wally a pleasant excursion and a break in our daily routine.

The "colored wing" usually held six black men and six black women. One of the women, jolly and heavyset, used to take walks around the grounds and would stop and chat with the women in my pavilion through the screen. Everybody liked her. When I was able to walk around, I would visit with her in the black pavilion. She kept goldfish in a bowl near her bed. She was the first black I ever knew personally.

There were two black men I was fond of, William and Maryland. Maryland wrote poems, and we traded. His were very different from mine, and I enjoyed reading them. One day he told me that he was dismissed and going home. I said, "Oh, I hope to be going home someday, too. If you ever come to my town, I hope you'll stop to see me."

"Where all do you live, Miss Margie?" he asked.

"In Hays."

"Oh, if I ever get to your town, I'll sure get a shuffle on!"

I did not know what he was talking about. Later I discovered that Hays at that time had laws forbidding Negroes to stay overnight within the city. The college was embarrassed by these discriminatory laws when staff invited Booker T. Washington to talk to the students. The college president discovered too late that their famous speaker was not welcome in any hotel in town. He declared that Washington would stay in his home on campus, then. The "authorities," whoever they were, told him his house was still within the city limits. Booker T. Washington ended up at the college farm outside the city.

There was a crafts shop in one building where patients could learn woodworking, leatherwork, weaving and other handcrafts. One woman was very gifted at soap carving. I still have in my cedar chest a baby in a bathtub, the baby's Ivory soap ringlets now turned to a faded gold. If no craft teachers were available, the patients taught each other.

Nina was older than I and had fought tuberculosis for most of her life. She had attended craft schools in Arizona and Colorado and shared her knowledge freely with others. She asked me to help her with orders for sewn and appliqued items from large department stores in Kansas City and Denver. She showed me how to do delicate hemstitching on appliques and how to make rolled hems on handkerchiefs. She even shared her design patterns with me, so I could start my own business after leaving the san, if I wanted. The baby dresses she made with miniature tucks and tiny roses were exquisite, and I hoped that I might have a child of my own someday to sew such dresses for.

Most of us attempted one way or another to earn money to supply our personal needs. One of the nurses offered to buy me a pair of pajamas if I would help her piece a flower garden quilt. She cut out the pieces, and I sewed them together. I was happy to feel useful as well as to have a new pair of pajamas.

Baggy pajamas hid a new development from me, however. When I was allowed to get up and exercise and to walk to the dining hall for my meals, I discovered that none of the dresses I'd brought with me to the san would fit. The "stringbean" of college days had gained weight while lying around in bed, like a cushioned cat on cream. Those were the only clothes I had. A friend from college days, Edith Mason, helped buy dresses and sleepwear for me and gave me mail order catalogs I could order from when I earned a little money.

Although I did some woodburning and other craftwork, it was my poetry hobby that continued to grow. Friends Etna and Alice showed me how to crimp the edges of a piece of plate glass and make a frame for my poems, using bright colored paints and aluminum foil in the background. By writing special verses for people for birthdays and holidays, I was able to earn a bit of spending money for postage. A few verses were printed in church bulletins and the *Aerend* magazine of the college. My verses were not modeled after the classic poems I had studied in literature classes, but after the homespun Edgar Guest verses that dealt with everyday experience.

Regular rest periods morning and afternoon were strictly

enforced every day. Lights had to be out at nine p.m. Many of my verses came to me in the silence of the airy nights. I learned to keep my letters and a pencil under my pillow. If a verse came to me in the night, I could write it on the envelope. Leaving the letters inside made the envelopes stiff enough to write on. With practice, I learned to move a finger to keep track of each line so that I didn't write words upon words in the dark.

The sanatorium was filled with patients much worse off than I. I tried to give friendship wherever I could and often surprised a lonely person with my original verses enumerating their good points to give them courage. Their gratitude fed my ego and made my days worth living. I sent poems and feature stories to newspapers in Kansas and Missouri. Occasionally one would be printed, and I'd receive a small check in the mail. It was always exciting to see an envelope from the *Kansas City Star.*

Soon I was receiving fan mail. People sent me stamps and money asking for copies of my verses. I was happy that when I was at Hays Protestant Hospital, my brother Charles had traded in my desk-style manual typewriter for a lightweight portable I could hold on my lap.

When Dr. Taylor found me typing copies of poems on it one day, he said that a little typing now and then might be permitted, but no heavy duty typing was allowed while I was on the rest cure.

My friends at Wesley Foundation at the college in Hays, under direction of Reverend Clare Van Metre and Cora Bibens, decided to help by publishing a collection of my poems. They sold enough advance copies to pay for the printing, and soon my book, "Through the Chinks at Life" was available. The title was from a poem "Walls Ter Chink" which I had written for my father about my childhood in our log house.

WALLS TER CHINK

Bestest time of all the year,
For us Ozark chillern here
Is the day in early fall
When we git ter chink the wall.

Folks in town have big board houses
Painted white in fancy stylsus;
Log 'uns bestest kind I think,
'Cause they've got some walls ter chink.

When there comes a cold ole day,
Ma says: "Boys, now quit yer play,
Hunt yer spades and git ter work
Diggin' up that red clay dirt."

Soon we've got enuf ter mix
Inter good ole mud what sticks;
Then we take some in a pan
And daub it on with jist our han'.

Pa won't let us use his trowel—
Says us kids too little now
Ter use machinery like that;
But we know where he keeps it at.
So maybe we can slip it down
When our Pa's nowhere aroun';
And then we'll do the job up right—
Fill them cracks all good and tight.

But anyway it's heaps of fun,
No matter how the daubin's done;
We're mighty lucky kids, I think,
Ter have a house with walls ter chink.

The book was well received by my friends and fans, and
the small edition sold well enough to give me much joy and a
little pin money.

Privacy for thinking and writing was hard to come by. I was
afflicted once with a new patient in the next bed who whined
constantly. One day we had cornbread on our trays. She held
her nose and said, "Pheuuu, what is wrong with this cornbread? It stinks like kerosene." I ate mine and found nothing
wrong, but as I glanced down the row of beds on the porch, I
saw all the empty trays with cornbread left uneaten. Another
day we had string beans. "Pheuuu, why do they always give us

these old beans? Don't they know I hate beans?" Again, the beans were left on all the trays. She made me so upset and nervous that I asked my doctor if I might walk down by the creek awhile to keep from going crazy.

He thought it unwise, as I would then be subject to juicy speculation about romance by the creek. He compromised by hanging a "Do Not Disturb" sign on my door.

I enjoyed a few minutes of quiet scribbling and decided this would do just fine. I was wrong. Other patients saw the sign and decided I must be sick. They sneaked around through other patient's rooms to get to me. They were sure I would want their company if I were sick, and they didn't want to neglect me. I took the sign down fast. Dr. Taylor once told me, "It's your friends that will kill you; your enemies will leave you alone."

Humor saved our sanity. Oddly enough, when I think of the sanatorium now, I hear laughter in the background.

Practical jokes were discouraged, but the men got away with one for a long time. They liked to initiate new male patients by giving them their first "electrical treatment." The man would be asked to lie flat on the floor. Then the others would run a vacuum sweeper up and down his back. It was supposed to remove the tubercle bacilli from his body.

I indulged in practical jokes myself, occasionally. Each of our beds had a metal sputum cup with a paper liner plus a paper sack pinned to the bed for our paper tissues. Every morning we had to spit into sputum cups for lab analysis. The technicians were checking for the rod bacilli that shows the presence of active tuberculosis. Although I had had hemorrhages, I never coughed up mucous and could never deposit anything more than saliva in the cups each morning. The labs could never find a TB germ in my contributions. Often the nurse would come back to have me try it again. This went on and on and on. One day I took some red embroidery floss, snipped a few little pieces into the sputum cup and spit on top of it. Several hours later the lab analyst, Miss Torgeson, came up to see me, highly amused. My sputum sample had had a number of heads bowed over the microscope that morning attempting to figure out what in the world was under that glass slide.

There were times when we resorted to gallows humor. We all looked forward to the day when we'd be well enough to be issued a permit to go shopping in town. There was a patient from the men's pavilion who was very ill in the hospital building, his body consumed by tuberculosis. For days the other patients had waited for word. He was dearly loved, and he had been in the hospital a long time. When one day we saw the long, black hearse pull out of the hospital driveway, we knew whom it was carrying. All of us had tears running down our cheeks, as we watched it slowly leave the gates of the san. Then one woman suddenly sat up in her bed and said, "Well! There is one patient who gets to go to town!" Our tears turned to laughter, and life—and death—went on.

Townspeople in Norton once protested against "Tuberks" coming into their city. They feared the spread of tuberculosis. Dr. Taylor gave the townfathers and mothers a talking-to, and assured them that Tuberks were trained to cover their mouths with tissue when they coughed, to wash their hands and not to spit on the street. "Hell, you're not going to catch TB from *my* patients," he said. "You'll get it from the old snorts in town who persist in spitting all over the street. Get yourself an ordinance about that, first!" We could always count on Dr. Taylor's sense of humor as well as his sense of fairness.

Once someone sent in a radio song dedication for "Annie," a little woman who not only suffered from tuberculosis but had so many scars she said her body resembled a Japanese battle field. Tuberculosis had ruined her throat until she could only whisper. The friend who had told Annie to listen for the dedication apparently did not select the song, or if he did, he had a macabre humor. As we all gathered around the radio, Annie was the first to break into laughter, as we heard the words, "We Are Going Down the Valley One by One."

The more freedom I had to walk around the grounds, the more mischief I was capable of getting into. The dairy farm at the sanatorium was fully equipped with everything needed to raise crops for the cows and convert their produce to milk, cream and butter for the patients. Once a rodeo came to perform for the patients, who watched and cheered from their porch windows. I was strolling on the grounds with another young woman at the time. Just as the rodeo performers were

51

leaving, two farmhands came along with a team of mules hitched to a wagon.

I asked them if I could drive their mules. They laughed and said, "Bet you can't drive 'em!" And I said, "Bet I can!" They didn't believe me at all, not knowing that I had ridden some of the oldest and most stubborn mules that ever existed to school as a child. Expecting that their mules wouldn't budge an inch for us, they let me climb in that wagon with the other girl. I clucked my tongue, said some Ozarkian magic words and drove that team of mules all around those big buildings. The people were still looking out of their windows and porches and thought we were part of the rodeo. Happily, Dr. Taylor didn't scold me.

Rest, mild exercise, good food and good humor built back my health. Towards the end of my rest cure, I began to hear more about an additional treatment that was beginning to be successfully practiced at the san. It was called pneumothorax and involved running a needle through the chest into the pleural lining. pumping in air and collapsing the lung. The basic idea of this treatment had been around since the 1800s, but greatly increased in popularity among physicians early in this century. Collapsing the lung and keeping it collapsed for one to three years did seem to retard or prevent further development of a tubercular lesion. Up to 50% of patients in some large institutions were treated with pneumothorax techniques into the 1940s, until the more effective anti-tuberculosis drug treatments became available.

Attendants would come to our pavilions on certain days and pick up patients in wheelchairs to take them to another building where the pneumothorax equipment was kept.

One day I had a call saying I was scheduled for pneumothorax. I felt there was some mistake, and I refused to go. Dr. Rarick had visited me that day, and he had said, "Now, Margie, you do what the doctors tell you to."

I still refused to go. Later I found out that the reason Dr. Cohen had asked me to come for pneumothorax was because he and Dr. Hall were fighting with each other over my porchmate, Neva. She was a gorgeous, sensuous redhead, and they were both smitten with her. Neva had been in Dr. Cohen's building for awhile before being transferred to Dr. Hall's pavilion. Now Dr. Cohen was inviting her to come for pneumothorax treatments, of which he was in charge. She told Dr. Cohen that she would take the pneumothorax treatments, "if Margie would."

Dr. Hall was in charge of my building. He hadn't scheduled me for pneumothorax treatment, consequently, I was in no hurry to have my lungs collapsed, just when they were nearly well.

When I asked Dr. Taylor why Dr. Cohen wanted me for pneumothorax, he stared at me. "My God..." he muttered and walked out. That was the end of pneumothorax for me and it was also the eventual end of Dr. Cohen.

I liked Dr. Cohen very much and was sorry to see him go. He used to bring his violin to our porches each Christmas and play carols for us. Once I asked him why, if he was Jewish, he played Christmas carols. "I play them for you, not me," was his swift reply.

Neva eventually took the pneumothorax treatments and continued them for a while after she was well enough to leave the sanatorium. She wrote me that her husband wondered how she would keep up the pneumothorax treatment once out of the san. "I really kidded him along," she wrote. "Told him, why, we'd just stop at a filling station like anybody else who needed a little air."

Finally, on a night in December of 1934, a nurse came to tell me to pack my trunk because Dr. Taylor had just called to say I would be dismissed early the next morning. A car would be waiting for me, and I was not to eat breakfast. It was a shock indeed. I did not even have a chance to tell my sanatorium friends goodby.

Hell, she's got a home!

SEVEN

A few days prior to my dismissal two members of the board of supervisors had come to the sanatorium to check on me. When they asked Dr. Taylor about me, he had said, "Oh, she's doing fine. She could be released, except she doesn't have a home to go to. If she has to go out and work full time, she'll probably have another breakdown. But if she had a home to go to, well, we could release her."

The supervisors went back to Hays, and one of them, Bill Phillips, happened to run into Jay D. Fellers on the street. "I hear you've been up to see Margie," Jay D. said, "How is she?"

The supervisor recounted Dr. Taylor's statements. Jay D. went home, talked to Bessie and called Dr. Taylor to ask if it were true. Then Jay D. said, "Hell, she's got a home to go to. Pack her trunk. We'll be there early, and tell her not to eat breakfast, we'll give her breakfast."

Bessie apologized for not having a room ready for me, but put me in their guest room which she always kept ready. I had only been there a few days when Jay D. put a round-trip bus ticket in my hand for Montier, Missouri. He said, "If I had a daughter that I hadn't seen for four years, I'd sure appreciate it if someone helped her come visit me."

That did not go for sisters. I stopped in Kansas City on my way to Montier. When Edna opened the door, she saw her formerly skinny sister plumped up 30 pounds heavier by the sanatorium's rich calcium diet and little exercise. She looked at me and laughed, "I knew all the time you weren't sick at all. You look as healthy as can be." That was her attitude toward me for several more years before she finally softened up.

It was good to see my dad again and to meet our new stepmother, Chloe Lee, a widow. We had encouraged Dad to marry again, as we knew how lonely he had been since Mother's death.

I had only been with them a couple days when the phone rang, and Jay D. told me to hurry back to Hays because the Farm Bureau wanted to hire me at their office.

There was no job, I found when I returned. It was just a trick to get me out of the cold, damp climate of the Ozarks before I caught cold.

Meanwhile, in the short time that I was away, Jay D. and Bessie had had their son, Edmond, and Jimmy Penrod, the hired man, repaper and paint a room for me. Bessie had sewn a peach-colored silk damask bedspread with nylon net over it. The boys had sawed out a kidney-shaped piece of wood for a dressing table top and painted it ivory. Bessie had "dolled it up," as she put it, with a skirt of the damask and net to match the bedspread.

When I saw that beautiful room, the tears began to flow. Bessie couldn't understand why I was crying. She wondered if I were disappointed with it all. It seemed to me a room fit for a princess, and I was so touched emotionally that for days I couldn't disturb that beautiful bed. I would wait each night until the family was asleep, then I would tiptoe into the hired girl's room and slip into bed with Fabiola who, like me, had grown up sharing sleeping quarters with many brothers and sisters.

Eagle-eyed Edmond became suspicious and told on me. It was difficult to explain my feelings when Bessie asked if something was wrong with my new bed.

I became now the daughter Bessie had always wanted before the tubercle bacilli had put an end to her childbearing years. Jay D. said there was only one thing wrong. When he had inquired about legally adopting me, he was told I was past the age for adoption. It was 1935; I was 27.

Halfway through his studies at K-State, Edmond had come home permanently from college. He was in love with Florence Tichenor, and they planned to be married in March. He believed he could learn what he needed to know on the farm from his father, and he was eager to begin modernization of their Higher View Dairy and to become a first class breeder of Holsteins. He did exactly that over the years, with much success, and at one time was president of the national Holstein organization. He was then, and still is, like a brother to me.

Bessie was a perfect housekeeper, but 1935 was the year for the first and worst dust storms ever known in Kansas. When the dust began to blow, Bessie covered everything she could with bedsheets. The dust was like sandpaper and could ruin the finish of furniture if brushed off carelessly with a cloth. When the wind went down, she would shake the sheets and start the laundry. She would vacuum all the furniture, wash all the windows and freshen the curtains. But then the wind would come up again, and it was all to do over.

The winds blew out crops and covered the sun with dust until days became darker than nights. Jay D. emerged from the bathroom one morning carrying a bucket of dirt he had brushed out of the tub. He jokingly asked, "Who in hell took a bath last night? They sure as Satan didn't clean that tub."

Laughter was the only way to save our sanity. The Fellers were masters at it despite all their troubles. When the storms were blowing and we cowered indoors, the men would play the women at cards to see who would cook the next meal. Often it was necessary to use an extra tablecloth to cover the table of food as we ate. It kept our plates clean as we reached under the cloth for each bite. Then Jay D. would shout, "Let's have a game of pinochle to see who washes the dishes!"

Dust settled so thickly on our arms it made a shower when brushed off. Once at the table, Jay D. raked his hand across my arm, and the dust blew. "My God," he said, "Don't you ever take a bath?"

When I left the sanatorium the nurses had given me an entire suitcase full of gauze face masks to wear in case I—or someone around me—had a bad cold. It looked to me like a lifetime supply. When the dust started to choke my breathing, I remembered those masks. The morning I walked in to breakfast wearing a white mask, Jay D. broke into uproarious laughter and teased me unmercifully. Over the next few hours, however, he watched my mask turn black with dust. "You got any more of those things?" he asked. Soon we were all sitting around in gauze masks playing pinochle.

One night in early spring Edmond sang for a community program in the Buckeye Township Hall. Bessie had sent his white suit to the cleaners, so he could properly usher in the springtime on stage. He looked handsome up there as he smiled and began to warble, "Rain, Rain, When You Gonna Rain Again, Rain." As he sang, we could hear the wind coming up outside. The dust sifted through the hall so quickly and so thickly we couldn't even see him by the time he'd finished. We spent most of the night there, waiting with others for the wind to slow down. When we finally set out for home, our car lights still could not penetrate the dusty darkness. One of the men stood outside on the car's running board, feeling for the mailboxes, so we'd know when to turn into our own driveway.

Jimmy and Edmond continued to milk the cows even though they couldn't save the milk. The dust turned it black before the white stream hit the buckets. This was long before Higher View Dairy acquired its automated dairy equipment.

One Sunday a truck driver pulled into our driveway to wait out a storm and parked directly in the path between barn and house. The dust was so dense that Jimmy and Edmond didn't see the truck in the path, and they bumped their heads when they made a fast dash for the house after milking.

The day no one laughed began with a phone call from Edmond to Florence, in which he learned of her little brother's illness. He hurried to be with Florence's family as they rushed the child to a hospital in Hays. They remained there all day, hoping the child might survive. He could not. His lungs were packed solid with dust which he had breathed while walking home from school during a dust storm.

With no winter wheat for pasture and no hay, the Fellers were forced to buy hay at high prices from out of state to feed their cows. The hay was of poor quality, and one by one, they watched their prize young heifers die. The veterinarian's post mortems showed stomachs full of thorny burrs, almost the only plants that would grow in Kansas during the drought, the only food the cows could scavenge besides the poor hay.

One day, as the vet drove away, the local minister drove in. While Edmond stood in the farmyard beside a dead calf, the minister reminded him that they were behind on their pledge to the church and that ministers had to eat, too. He suggested that produce was as good as money. He meant well, but Edmond was thinking of the milk he was forced to dump on the ground, the few eggs they were getting, the dead calves and no promise of crops. He knew how much his parents loved the church and how proud they had always been to support it. He understood how much this visit would embarrass them. Yet, he didn't mince words when he faced the preacher and sent him away empty-handed.

Bessie was hurt when she found out what Edmond had said to their pastor. Yet the truth was obvious. There was little left to go around. I was worried, too, for I knew I had been, and still was, an extra expense for them during this critical time. I wanted to work. I had heard about WPA jobs, and so I applied in Hays for an opening for a teacher of wood crafts for children. The bureaucrat in charge complained that I didn't have a college degree, but supervisor Bill Phillips came to my rescue and advised him that sometimes experience was the best teacher and that I had studied crafts at the sanatorium.

So I soon had my first part-time job, training children to use small jigsaws to cut plywood into animal shapes for bookends and toys.

I was given a corner in a WPA mattress factory to store my supplies. When I overheard women employees talking about clothing shipments to the factory and how they got first choice, I wondered about the fairness of it all. One morning I was told that the WPA director was in the hospital. Men from the "Square Dealers Club" had tossed him down the stairs for not giving them whatever it was they had demanded.

That did it for me. I had known too many needy people who were thankful for any help they received. I couldn't understand those who demanded a "square deal" beyond that. From then on I refused to stand in line with those people when our WPA checks were handed out. The office either had to mail mine or give it to me privately. I was embarrased by the WPA job even though I enjoyed working with the children, and I definitely needed the money.

I walked the streets searching for another job. In restaurants, I would offer to work for my board. When a new doctor came to Hays, I hurried to apply for a receptionist position. He told me he had just hired someone, but I could do him a great favor by sitting in front of his window for awhile. Then passersby might think he had a client. Must have helped. Five years later, when he delivered my first baby, he had built up a huge practice.

I was very happy when I was able to pay for a room once again at Mrs. Barry's rooming house. I hadn't been there long before I began to find small cartons of cottage cheese and pint boxes of milk at my door. I called the L. K. Dairy, owned by Lou and Katie Krause, to tell them the delivery boy had made a mistake, as I hadn't ordered anything. "It's no mistake," they assured me. "It was just a surplus. It would spoil if we didn't give it away. And don't worry about it. There's no charge." They obviously were well aware of the place dairy products held in a "Tuberk's" diet.

Finally, I found a full-time job at the college's agricultural experiment station, where my father and my younger brother John had earlier worked. Mr. Aicher, the director, dreaded writing up his annual reports and was happy to have me write them, along with many other jobs that exercised my journalistic skills. "I know you're of good stock," he said. "Your dad cultivated our black walnut test orchard with the mule team. Of all the men I've hired, he was the only one who could outwalk those spirited mules."

My younger brother had worked at the experiment station until he had broken down with tuberculosis, at roughly the same time as I had. He had been cared for by his friends in Hays and then went home to stay with our dad in Montier for a while until he recovered.

John had always had health problems. Mother contracted erysipelas just after his birth. Her breasts turned purple. He caught erysipelas, too, and nearly died. He was, in fact, pronounced dead by the doctor. My dad refused to believe that John was dead. He wrapped a sugar cube in a bit of cloth and put it in the baby's mouth. He held him a long, long time, and finally John started sucking on the sugar cube. Gradually, he recovered, but later on in his childhood he had typhoid and just about every disease available to kids. He had trouble with his legs when he was in high school. He also fell into what the rest of us considered bad company and took up smoking. But he survived everything, married, had two children and lived into his seventies.

Some of John's best times were when he was working at the experiment station in Hays. Some of mine were, too.

The Dish Washer

EIGHT

The dust storms had finally ceased and the experiment station was trying to figure out how to prevent them from rising again. There was much for dry-land farmers to learn about how to keep their soil from blowing, and I helped to write up the pamphlets of information.

Mr. Aicher had no love for what he termed "suit case farmers." After the Depression many Kansas farms ended up in the hands of eastern bankers or insurance agencies. Their hired farm managers did not always have the good of the farmland uppermost in their minds, and many of them were barely familiar with western Kansas farming. Everyone, newcomers as well as old-timers, had to learn new ways of farming the land.

Along with teaching farmers to fallow their land properly, the machine shop workers at the experiment station invented new agricultural machines such as the dam-lister, which helped to hold the water on the fields. Plows equipped with the dam-lister threw up little dams just a few feet apart in the lister row and thus caught and held the water.

I was intrigued with the newly invented hopper-dozer. Mr. Aicher let me ride along to watch it work. Grasshoppers were so numerous they stripped alfalfa fields like a biblical plague. The hopper-dozer had an aluminum vat full of crank case oil on the front of a sturdy tractor. As the dozer pushed its way across the fields, swarms of startled grasshoppers would fly up, hit the backboard and fall into the oil. After several runs across the field, the driver would stop and with a perforated shovel remove the dead hoppers from the oil, leaving them in a stack at the edge of the field. By the end of the season, there was a huge stack of dry, dead, well-oiled grasshoppers at the edge of the experiment station's alfalfa field. The grasshoppers were full of moisture, and it had taken weeks of hot Kansas sun to dry them out so they could be burned.

There was a rustic night club on land adjacent to the alfalfa field. It was a lovely entertainment spot with trees, very popular for outdoor dances under the stars. The action sometimes strayed from the dance floor, however, and Mr. Aicher had been troubled by the amount of paraphernalia he'd found in his field, left by lovelorn patrons who'd wandered away from the club.

His chance came on a lovely summer night. A famous dance orchestra had been advertised for the club's outdoor pavilion, and a large crowd had gathered. The wind was just right, and so were the hoppers. Mr. Aicher asked one of his men to set fire to the stacks. When the fragrance of roasting grasshoppers wafted across the dance floor, the dancers quickly departed. The club lost a lot of money and soon closed.

Mr. Aicher used a camera to illustrate the ingenious inventions of the experiment station and how they could be used by farmers in the fields. He decided to turn the dark room over to me to manage the developing and printing of his films, and I was pleased to add a new skill to my working repertoire.

I was happy in Hays at Mrs. Barry's rooming house. Her husband was not well, and so she took in boarders to supplement their income. Her boarders at that time included several single business people, a few students and teachers from the college, some WPA engineers and me. We all enjoyed her home cooking.

One day she confided to me that she had a new dishwasher coming. In those days, a dishwasher walked on two legs. She asked me to help the new arrival get acquainted, for she wanted him to like his new job. Dishwashers were hard to find.

I promised to do my best, but I was not too interested in the fellow when he arrived, as he was not only an inch beneath my 5' 10" height, he was eight years younger. Besides, I was mooning over another young man at the time, one who had strong religious convictions. Nevertheless, the dishwasher did begin to pester me for dates, which I refused.

I did enjoy chatting with him, however. When he returned

for his second year in college and continued to ask me out, he argued that as long as we enjoyed each other's company, why should age or anything else enter in?

I remembered then an odd theory that Dr. Taylor had proffered when I complained to him once that it always seemed as if short men were enamored with me, rarely a tall one. "It's nature's way of keeping the human race from getting too long in the chest," he said. "TB seems to like long chests. Count your children lucky if they get a father shorter than you are." I wasn't pleased with the advice.

A circus came to Hays for one day, and I wanted to go. But my boyfriend refused. His religion didn't approve of using captive animals for entertainment.

When John Sutcliffe heard that bit of boarding house gossip, he came looking for me and said, "Come on, I'll take you."

I retorted, "You little shrimp, you couldn't take me anywhere." We happened to be standing at the top of the stairs. *Gone With the Wind* had not yet been filmed, yet my admirer, whose ears stuck out somewhat like Clark Gable's, swept me up in his arms and carried me downstairs, and we went to that circus. John had a little money saved from painting house numbers on curbs, but it turned out we didn't even need to pay admission. We got lost and somehow entered the circus from the rear, passing mangy camels and half-naked women in dressing rooms as we tried to find the entrance. By the time we'd found it, we were in free.

On the way home, we climbed up in a treehouse above the sidewalk and listened to the conversations of circusgoers as they strolled home. I didn't know anyone quite like this.

We certainly did enjoy our times together, and four years later, on October 28, 1939, we were married.

A few days before the ceremony, we went to Norton and had Dr. Taylor check my health. I was doing fine. He checked out my prospective husband, too. As John was standing behind the fluoroscope, Dr. Taylor peered closely at the screen and pronounced, "He still has his heart, Marjorie. He may have given it to you, but thank goodness, he still has it."

The marriage license cost John $4.00. After celebrating our Golden Wedding in 1989, he assured me that I had been a pretty good bargain.

We moved to his family farm near Park, Kansas, to live with his widowed father. John had studied animal husbandry and art at Hays, but allergies to animals, pollens and especially relatives in close confinement convinced him after a year or so to go back to school.

With our first daughter, Judy, born in 1941, we moved to Manhattan, Kansas, where John entered the veterinary college. It was during wartime, housing was hard to come by and we felt very fortunate to rent a pleasant, two-story frame house with a coal furnace in the basement and guinea hens in the yard. It was across the street from the college dairy where John milked cows to help pay his way through college.

One day during a dismal rain there was a knock at the door. A wraith walked straight in and past me to an empty chair. Later she explained that God had sent her. She was tired, and the chair was empty. Her coat was wet, wrinkled and flecked with black and white lint. Her hair was awry, and her face of sixty-some years was wrinkled. I did not like her and stood staring.

"Mr. Howenstine tells me you have two rooms you are not using," she said. "We'll need both of them," she announced. "Charley's new job starts tomorrow."

That was that. Charley, her husband, started work as a janitor at the college the next day, and she packed their belongings into the two small rooms.

They were a memorable couple. Charley was late to work one morning and couldn't find his false teeth. He gulped down his bacon and eggs and tried to drink his coffee. Not one to complain, he drank it all before he confessed to Alice that it hadn't tasted quite right.

"Charley!" she said, "Where did you leave your teeth last night?"

"In a cup by the wash basin," he answered.

"Oh, Charley," she said, "you have drunk your teeth!" In her hurry to make coffee for him in the dark, she'd used that cup to dip water from the bucket, and the teeth must have fallen in and melted. They were cheap plastic mail-order teeth. Happily, he could order another pair from the same place.

Alice caught cold once from picking strawberries in the rain to help a truck farmer bring in his crop. She reported that her old doctor told her she had "asthma in her barnacles." Otherwise, she was full of boundless energy and kindness.

Situated as we were at the outskirts of Manhattan, we were continually presented with unwanted kittens. With the coming of Alice and Charley Rice, the kittens multiplied. Stray dogs began to arrive to scrap over leftovers and bones on our front lawn. Alice brought a female Persian inside, and it yowled its heart out. She finally consented to having it spayed and allowed the "poor homeless creature" to recover on top her bed while she slept on the floor beside it!

Any helpless being received her aid and love. Neighbor children whose mothers worked were often fed from her table. She bought them toys. She played endless, make-believe games with my three-year-old daughter and talked for her dolls.

Once Judy's new oilcloth Easter rabbit got lost. She refused to go to sleep without it. Her screams grew louder as we lost patience. We could not find it. Alice came with Charley and his flashlight to help us search. They were both in long, white nightgowns and made a spectacular scene in the darkness. They returned emptyhanded. Alice comforted Judy by saying, "Auntie Rice couldn't find that rabbit, but God knows where it is, and it will be safe. Auntie Rice will pray, and God will tell her in the morning where to find it."

As John and I were getting our breakfast next morning, Alice walked past us as if in a trance, still wearing that long, white gown. We watched from the window as she walked straight into the garden, bent over and picked up that rabbit from under a cabbage leaf.

When I became pregnant with my second child, my husband was encamped in the local army barracks while continuing his schooling (the Army needed veterinarians), and I was nauseated with morning sickness. I wondered how I would survive the pregnancy.

But there stood Alice in the bedroom door. "You just stay right there in bed. I'll fix breakfast for Judy and care for her. Don't you know if you stay off your feet that sickness will go away? You just stay right there and I'll bring your meals."

The long months of pregnancy and separation from my husband while he was in the service were only endurable because of her kindness.

By the time John was out of the Army and ready to graduate, our baby Juanita was crawling. Alice offered to babysit while Judy and I went to his graduation. When we returned to the old house with the January wind whipping at its windows, we found the interior a shambles. Furniture was pulled out, magazines were strewn about, rugs were twisted, cupboards and drawers were emptied and their contents tossed on the floor. Towels, washcloths, soap were thrown into the tub. Shoes and socks were all over the bedroom, toys were tossed out of their box and my lovely asparagus fern lay uprooted with its beautiful pot that my husband had bought for me lying broken on the floor beside it.

Juanita sat in the middle of the floor exploring an upside down doll buggy. Crouched in a corner was Alice Rice. Her knees were red and scraped.

"I'm sorry about everything," she cried. "I'm sorry about the plant. I tried to keep her from breaking anything, but she pulled it off so quick I couldn't catch it. I watched so she didn't put things in her mouth. She cried all the time she was in her crib. I couldn't bear to hear her cry. I tried rocking her but it didn't work, so I just turned her loose and crawled with her. My knees hurt, but she was happy."

"Well," I thought, "too bad the kid isn't old enough to remember this. She'll never have a day like this again."

Alice Rice was the closest thing to a grandmother we ever had for our children, and it was hard to leave her behind when the new veterinarian began looking for a place to set up his practice.

The Cows

NINE

Audubon, Iowa, was a small rural town of 2,800 people. It was surrounded by rolling green hills, lush fields and farmsteads every half mile or so, each one a picturesque grouping of a white, two-story wood-frame house on a green lawn, with a rambling red barn nearby, plus a machine shed, hog house, chicken house and a few other outbuildings.

Farmers in this part of western Iowa were relatively prosperous, and they raised corn, oats, alfalfa, cattle, hogs, dairy cows and a few chickens. The responsibilities of my veterinarian husband in this countryside included the state-mandated vaccination of hogs for hog cholera and the state-required testing of cows, both beef and dairy, for tuberculosis.

Every single cow in every herd in Audubon County had to be tuberculin tested at least once a year until the herd was certified three times in a row as TB free. By law, any cow that tested positive had to be slaughtered. Beef cattle had to be certified free of tuberculosis before they could be moved across county or state lines to be sold for steak and hamburger. Dairy cows had to be free of tuberculosis before their milk could be sold. Cows had to be tested before going to a county or state fair. John's rapidly growing large animal practice included a hefty amount of TB testing.

By 1946, most every farmer and dairyman had gotten used to frequent TB testing. They understood more or less why it had to be done and did not protest. My husband said that, in fact, the Federal Bovine Tuberculosis Eradication Program had been a godsend for some farmers during the Depression, as the government paid them for reactors that had to be slaughtered, and they didn't have enough money to feed the cows anyway or enough customers with money to buy.

But in 1931 there had been riots in Cedar County, Iowa, against compulsory tuberculin testing. A thousand, steamed-up people prevented animal health officials from conducting tuberculin tests on a farm and created a hullaballoo that lasted several days.

It is easy to understand why some cattle owners objected to tuberculin testing. The rules were simple: if a cow reacted positively to the test, it had to be slaughtered. And a good many reactors looked perfectly healthy. Some folks could only see their beef and milk money going down the drain.

What they couldn't see was the *Mycobacterium bovis,* the bacillus causing tuberculosis in cattle. It was a very close relative of *Mycobacterium tuberculosis,* the invader of humans. Too close a relative, in fact. The ancient Greek physicians had known that tuberculosis infected cattle as well as humans and suspected some relationship. But only later on, towards the turn of the 20th century, when scientists finally were able to trap the critters in their microscopes, did they discover that both the bovine and human type of bacillus could and did live in both hosts.

That meant that cattle could spread the disease to humans and vice versa. It could be spread from cows to humans by contact and through infected milk and meat. An infected human working with cattle could infect the animals.

There were a lot of tuberculous cattle early in this century. There were, in fact, a frightful number of them, perhaps 25 to 50% of the bovine population. They were everywhere.

No wonder so many children in the late 1800s and early 1900s contracted the primary TB infection. They were susceptible to bacilli floating around in their homes and schools, bacilli that came from actively infectious adults. In addition, they drank cow's milk, unpasteurized, which frequently came from tuberculous cows. If they lived on farms, they may have been in physical contact with diseased cows while they did the "chores" of milking, feeding and cleaning. Infection from the bovine type of tuberculosis was most often found in children, where the bacilli attacked glands, bones and intestinal membranes.

My husband told me of one farm woman who had become very angry when John told her that her milk cow had tested positive and must be destroyed. "That's my baby's only milk!" she protested.

Happily, both medical scientists and veterinarians were equally curious early on about the workings of this strangely insidious disease. They were able to test many of their theories about TB in cattle through experiments and autopsies, something they could not do freely with human subjects.

When the tuberculin test was introduced around the turn of the century, it was the certainty everyone had been looking for. Over and over, the veterinarians and researchers were able to show that if an animal tested positive, it was harboring tuberculosis bacteria, no matter how healthy it appeared on the hoof, no matter if none of its excretions showed presence of *M. bovis*. And if it had the primary infection, then it could later develop the reinfection phase, the acute contagious phase, which might manifest as a hacking cough with a cheesy material coughed up, with gradual emaciation and death of the animal. Very like a human victim.

The veterinarians could do what doctors could not. If an animal tested positive, they could kill it and search its tissues to see where the tubercles were located. They were always present, no matter how robust the animal. All that a human doctor could do was warn his positive-testing patient to have frequent X-rays and not overdo. If a breakdown ensued, he could quarantine his patient in a sanatorium and hope that time and nature would put the infectious disease into remission.

Though the first response from farmers and dairy men was often shock and anger at the prospect of having to slaughter large numbers of their herds, most realized that it was the only solution in the long run. The goal was a 100% tuberculosis-free bovine population for our country.

In the United States, the federal government was involved quite early in the 1900s in setting up quarantine stations in U.S. ports, and eventually in the countries that exported cattle here, particularly the United Kingdom. Incoming cattle were TB tested, thus assuring clean imports to this country. Within our borders, the states and counties, cooperating with the federal government, started testing and keeping records. Cattle couldn't be shipped across state and county lines without TB testing. Herd accreditation and accreditation of counties and states was another control mechanism.

Within a very short span of years, due to stringent enforcement of TB testing of cattle and slaughter of all that tested positive, the tuberculosis bacillus was almost eradicated from the bovine population of the United States. The year 1935 was the largest ever for tuberculin testing, with millions of cattle tested. By the end of the year, 22 states were listed as modified accredited areas, and 79.1% of all counties in the nation had achieved this rating.

By the time my veterinarian husband started TB testing in Audubon, the major campaign was past. The wholesale slaughter of thousands of infected animals in previous years had resulted in a surviving population of healthy animals, relatively free of the ancient scourge.

Testing continued and still continues, because the presence of even one infected animal, if neglected, leads to rapid exposure of the non-reactors.

Federal meat inspection and federal legislation mandating pasteurization of milk were new laws that protected our children even further from the possibility of exposure to tainted meat or milk. In our little town, John would put on his official white coveralls whenever he got a call from the local butcher and would go down to the meat market and inspect the hanging carcass and the severed head of whatever cow had been killed that day. John always had me cook his roast beef extremely well done, nevertheless, and he would never touch rare meat. He had contracted brucellosis or undulant fever himself as a boy, from drinking raw milk.

When it was learned that heating milk would destroy tuberculosis bacilli, it became a compulsory measure in many areas. In the pasteurization process, milk is heated to 147° F., held there for 30 minutes, then chilled at 50° F. or lower until ready to be used. Chicago in 1911 was the first city to mandate pasteurization, followed by New York in 1915. Wherever pasteurized milk replaced raw milk consumption, the incidence of tuberculosis went down, particularly in children.

As with everything else, a few people resisted pasteurization, and there are still people today who prefer to drink raw milk. I always feel that they take the lives of their children in their hands. They do not know who is testing the cows. Pasteurization is such an easy, simple solution.

With the enormous success of TB testing of cows and the eradication of positive reactors in beef and dairy herds, and with the banning of sales of raw milk, the incidence of TB infection of children dropped dramatically. In 1926 Minnesota grade-school children showed a 47.3% positive reaction to the tuberculin test. In the same schools in 1954,it was down to only four percent.

My own children were never allowed to drink raw milk or eat rare meat. They were among the first generations of children in the world, probably all through recorded time, to grow up with minimal exposure to the tuberculosis bacillus, due to near-eradication of TB in cattle and to the lessening exposure to primary human TB sources because of the quarantine effected by the sanatoria.

But danger was lurking in our new home. We had our veterinary office in our little house on a corner of Davenport Street in Audubon. I was not only wife and mother, but housekeeper, laundress, office manager, receptionist, mixer of medicines, printer of medicine labels, bookkeeper and bill collector.

Judy was five and Juanita was one when we started in business. Dr. Taylor had told me before I married that I could have one child. "Having the babies won't kill you, but caring for them will," he had advised. He'd also had some advice about housecleaning: "Don't worry about the dust, because as long as it's settled, it won't get in your lungs." But I worried about it anyway, and I tried to keep the office and house spick and span as well as keeping the children clean, happy and well-fed.

John did well at his work, and after our first six months, he surprised me by hiring a young farm woman to help with the cleaning. With two rambunctious children to care for and office calls to handle, he wanted to make sure I didn't overdo.

But he was a little too late.

Sleepless Nights

TEN

One lovely summer Sunday we went to Sunday School and church and then had lunch at a local cafe. Back at home, I put the children to bed for their naps, and we decided to rest a while, too, since both of us had recently had the flu, and then we'd go for a drive in the lovely countryside around Audubon.

We had rested only a short time when suddenly I began to cough. The old tubercle bacillus reared its ugly head once again as great mouthfuls of foamy blood came up from my lungs. John had never witnessed a hemorrhage before and was thoroughly frightened. He phoned the elderly town physician, Dr. Jensen. The doctor peered at me from the doorway of our bedroom, shaking his head, and told us that he had never seen a case like this in all his years of practice, and he didn't know what to do.

I assured him that I did know, and I had already removed the pillow from under my head. I had him phone Dr. Taylor at the Norton sanatorium. Dr. Taylor told him that I should lie quietly for a week or more, and then he wanted to see an X-ray to compare with those still on file at the san. He also said that perhaps I should return to the sanatorium because of the danger to my children.

When John went to pick up the X-ray, Dr. Jensen told him he was sorry, but the TB had spread all over both lungs. John was scared, but I explained to him that regular doctors were not trained to read X-rays for TB, and I was sure that he was wrong. Later I asked Dr. Taylor what Dr. Jensen had seen all over both lungs. He laughed and said, "It was probably the gas from that baked potato you'd eaten the night before."

He could find no significant difference in the old and new X-rays. He said that the same dime-sized tubercle located in the apex of my right lung had erupted again, causing the adjacent blood vessel to overflow.

In July of 1946, back to the sanatorium I went. Mr. McFadden, our local undertaker, took me in his ambulance. Lying beside him as he drove and looking up into his face, I knew he felt sorry for me. "You know, I'm mighty lucky," I asserted. "Not many folks have a chance to talk to their undertaker when he takes them on trips."

I was taken to a room in a big new building at the sanatorium, several stories high. There were no porches, just regular windows. This stay at the san was very different from the previous one. With my husband and two babies left behind, it was heartbreaking for me as well as for them.

It was particularly hard on John to take care of the children and maintain his fledgling veterinary practice at the same time. He and the wife of an older veterinarian in Audubon tried to find a housekeeper, but none were available. John even considered giving up his promising new practice and taking a government job in Omaha. He called his sister who was living on a farm in western Kansas to see if she could take care of our two girls. "Sure," she said, "I'll just turn 'em loose with all the other wild turkeys." Meaning her six kids. They were all living in a basement at the time, as they hadn't built their house yet.

Happily, before John went too far, Emmert Fiscus knocked at the door one night. "You the new doc?" he asked. He said he had a girlfriend who wanted to come to Audubon, and he wondered if John might need some help. He certainly did.

I was happy to know that my children were being cared for, yet I missed them so much that I had difficulty in choking back the tears. One day a nurse noticed my girls' photos on my dresser. She told me that hers were about that age when she first came to the san as a patient. But her husband got tired of waiting for her and married the housekeeper. She had never seen the children again and in fact had never gone home again. She just stayed on as a nurse.

I couldn't sleep that night, and I soon learned that many of the nurses at the san had had the same experience. Also, many of the men who worked there had come as patients, and when they could not support the families they left at home, their wives had married other men who could. The tubercle bacillus was a home-breaker in more ways than one.

It also was very tough on the medical profession. Until health professionals began to understand how extremely infectious tuberculosis was, a disgracefully high percentage of young nursing and medical students started their schooling with negative TB tests and ended as positive reactors. It was a dangerous disease for everyone involved.

John wrote and telephoned often, but when he told me how wonderful the new hired girl was, helping with the housework and children and managing his calls—she even canned the string beans from our garden—I felt terrified and useless. What I could not see was that his wavy brown hair was turning prematurely gray from worrying about me.

He did not tell me that the hired girl gave the wrong medicine to a man with a sick cat, enough to kill half the cats in the county. Nor that when John requested the man's name, the girl said she didn't ask it as he'd paid cash. And when he learned she'd overcharged him as well, he knew he had lost that client for sure.

Night after night I could not go to sleep, wondering what was happening at home. I would finally drop off from sheer exhaustion, and then my nerves would jerk me awake again. July, August and most of September dragged by like this. I still had not seen Dr. Taylor, the sanatorium superintendent who had been so kind to me twelve years ago. I couldn't understand why he didn't come to see me. One sleepless night I decided to write him a letter that I planned to mail in the morning.

Early next morning I awoke to find him standing in my doorway. He said, "I had a dream last night. I dreamed you were in trouble, so I hurried into my car and was coming to help you. I came to a big rock in the middle of the road that I couldn't get around. I got out and lifted that God-damned car right over the rock, and then I woke up."

He assured me that he could find no damage to my lung, but because of the children, it was best for me to stay away awhile. He said he was leaving for Topeka on business and would check on me when he returned.

Later that day I heard a rumor that he had gone to lobby the Kansas legislature. He was so determined to wipe out tuberculosis that he had sponsored a bill to legalize the removal of anyone diagnosed with TB to a desert island or other isolated place, much like a leper colony.

That night I fell asleep long enough to dream that I was in a rat maze trying to find my way out. Round and round I ran, and when I finally reached the exit, there stood my husband with a baseball bat saying, "You can come home when Dr. Taylor says you can."

The dream haunted me all the next day, and I feared falling asleep that night. But when exhaustion finally pulled me under, I dreamt that I was in a deep, dark pit. Again and again I tried to clamber up the wet, slippery sides. I gave up to rest on the bottom and then noticed a slender spider web dangling in front of me. I reached for it but turned it loose—no such slender thread could hold my weight. But it held my attention, and soon I reached up and began to climb it as I had watched our Judy climb the rope that dangled from our maple tree. I was out of the pit as I awoke. That slender thread must have been what was left of my faith in God. Prayers had helped before and might again.

The next day when the French doctor who was in charge of patients in my section made his rounds, he told me that he'd decided to dismiss me.

"I know why you can't sleep," he said. "I was at Dunkirk... You won't get well unless you sleep, and you won't sleep until you're home." He explained that research showed the tuberculosis bacilli could not be carried more than twenty feet through the air from a cough. I had no cough, they had never found a TB germ on me and, if I would promise to stay twenty feet away from my children, never let my dishes out of my room and sterilize any sewing I did by hanging it in direct sunlight for six hours, then I could go home.

I always wondered if Dr. Taylor had told the French doctor to release me before he left for Topeka to lobby for his proposed legislation. I was gone before he returned. That was the last time I saw Dr. Taylor or heard from him. The bill did not pass. Dr. Taylor died within a short time after that, much too young.

For most of the next year in our home in Audubon, I lived in a back bedroom away from the children. There was a small throw rug positioned exactly twenty feet away where they could stand and talk to me. Judy could now share her kindergarten songs with me and tell me the news of the neighborhood. But in the three months I was at Norton, Juanita had nearly forgotten me. She would stand on the rug and look at me as if I were some strange creature and then run. How my arms ached to hold her.

Most of each day I rested in my room. The hired girl would bring a plate of food, scrape it off onto my private plate and take the first plate back to the kitchen. I had a small electric burner to heat water for washing my dishes. I had my own commode. If I did any sewing, knitting or crocheting for the children, it was hung on the clothesline in the sun all day.

I was happy to be home. I could answer the telephone and take my husband's calls. I could do his bookwork.

But I could also worry about things over which I had no control. Dr. Taylor had told me of the dangers of infection from TB germs on shoe soles because of people who spat on public streets. Although ordinances against spitting were instituted across the U.S. in the early 1900s with good results, it did not entirely wipe out this unhealthy and disgusting habit.

Audubon had no nursing home in those days to care for the elderly and infirm. Dear old Mr. Riley was taken in by a compassionate widow at the end of our block. He was no longer able to work, and his only interest in life was to walk uptown each morning to be with the "boys," other old men like himself who had nothing else to do.

Mr. Riley had just enough steam to make it from his house to the slight hill outside my window before he needed to stop and cough. Every morning he coughed up great mouthfuls of ugly mucous and spat it upon our sidewalk or the grass alongside. The lawn outside my window was a favorite spot for my children to play, and it was hard to keep them from congregating there. I listened to their laughing voices and hoped that the French doctor who had told me that sunshine would kill the bacilli was right.

My education in communicable diseases continued with the introduction of a new hired girl who came to the door of my room one day. "Well, I got even with him," she crowed. "I married his son." She mentioned one of the town fathers. "When I first moved here, he tried to chase me out of town because of my syphilis. I just wanted to get even with him, so I got his son drunk and married him. His father made us get annulled, but at least I slept with him all night!"

Here I was, hiding away in a back room to protect my children from tuberculosis, and this woman was supposed to be taking care of them?

As usual, John shook his head and said that hired girls were hard to find. The next one merely had trench mouth, which we only discovered after she'd been cooking for the girls a few weeks. Luckily, they didn't catch it.

For a time, in between the hired girls, John's sister Elizabeth, a Red Cross disaster nurse, came to take care of our daughters. We had always taught Judy to be self-sufficient. She was allowed to take baths by herself in the washtub, and we felt that it was more important that she learn to do things by and for herself than that she be impeccably clean. Judy's "Aunt Itt" was used to ordering around cadres of nurses during hurricanes, but her authoritarian tactics directed toward Judy's bathing methods brought only screams and yells.

This was not the only battle between the two of them. One evening at supper Judy had finished eating and put her dishes in the sink. Then she decided she wanted something more and asked for a spoon. Elizabeth said, "Oh, here, use mine." Judy began to scream, "No, my mommy always washes spoons first. No dirty spoons!" Impressed, Elizabeth got up and ran some water from the tap over the spoon and handed it back to Judy. More screams. "Momma always washes spoons with soap and water and rinses them in hot water!"

I do not know what emotional effect my quarantine had on my daughters, and they have virtually no memories of these times to draw on. But I do remember one summer evening when Judy had been playing at a neighbor girl's house. We had always told the children to come back home when it was dark. Our trust that they would do so was generally rewarded with good behavior. Just as darkness was beginning to settle over the trees that I could see from my window, I heard Judy's light footsteps running up the sidewalk. Then I heard her throw herself into the iris bed beneath my window and sob as if her little heart would break.

After nine months of this I was well again and resumed normal life with my family. But I kept my dishes separate from theirs for many more years. Tuberculosis is a silent killer that sneaks in when least expected. Whenever I finished a meal, I put my dishes in a steel pan and boiled them, unwashed, on the stove, before washing them separately from the others. They did not have the sparkle of the other dishes, but they certainly were sterile.

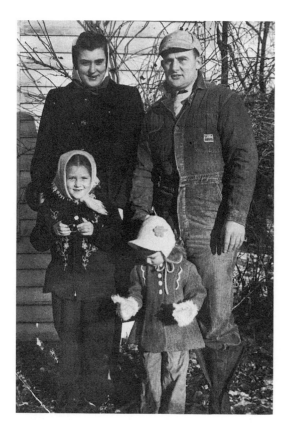

Marjorie McVicker Sutcliffe with Dr. John W. Sutcliffe, Judy and Juanita, about 1947.

The Miracle Drugs

ELEVEN

That wasn't the end of TB for me, however. The bacillus struck again two years later, in 1948, with another slight hemorrhage as warning. I went right back to bed.

But this time there was something new in the world. A drug called streptomycin. It was first produced in 1945 by S. Waksman and fellow researchers. It was the first drug in history able to reverse the potentially lethal course of the tuberculosis bacterium. Initially it was tried on guinea pigs and shortly after on humans.

Dr. Merselis wanted to try it on me, too. For forty days John took me to the doctor's office each morning and evening for streptomycin. In the morning the shots were given in my left hip and right arm. In the afternoon, the right hip and left arm. The rest of the day I stayed in my room, resting in bed.

During the summer this was going on, one of my Ozark nieces came to live with us, while she worked in the fields detasseling corn. Her mother, my brother Bob's wife, worried about Genevieve catching TB from me and let me know how concerned she was. While I was boiling my dishes and staying away from people, Genevieve's younger sister at home on their Missouri farm was allowed to play frequently at the home of a neighbor girl whose father was dying with TB. Most likely the family knew nothing about the tubercle bacilli, and no doubt the water bucket had a dipper from which they all drank, just as my Ozark family had done in my childhood days.

Faye, the daughter at home, later came down with TB, the only one of my parents' sixteen grandchildren to get the disease. She was taken to the Missouri sanatorium where surgery was performed on her lung. Prior to 1945, lung surgery for tuberculosis involved removal of an entire lung or separate lobes. But in that year E. A. Boyden at the University of Minnesota demonstrated that a small area of diseased tissue could be removed, leaving the remainder of the lung intact and functioning. That worked for Faye.

The streptomycin, happily, worked for me. It is now 1991 and I have had no more setbacks since taking the shots 45 years ago. Soon after streptomycin was produced in 1946, J. E. Lehman presented para-aminosalycylic acid or PAS, which also had a suppressive effect on the tubercle bacilli. In 1951, W. Fox introduced isoniazid. The latter remains among the four main drugs in use today: isoniazid, rifampin, PZA and ethambutol.

And the word remains control, not cure. The drugs kill most of the bacteria, but there is always the chance that the drugs may not succeed in finding every last little bacterium, just as there is also the possibility that the bacteria may mutate to a resistant form. Periodic examinations are recommended as long as a person reacts to tuberculin.

There is, unfortunately, no vaccination for tuberculosis. Over the years, researchers have produced several times what they thought to be a vaccination material. But with further study, the vaccination substance was always shown to be more dangerous than the disease. All we have is prevention and control.

Every year the state mobile X-ray unit from the National Tuberculosis Association came to Audubon to check me out. They had me on their list, among others in town. My children were checked as well, though they had tuberculin tests, not X-rays, as it was felt that X-rays were not good for children. The schools did tuberculin tests, too, though I don't know if that was through the county health department or in conjunction with the Tuberculosis Association. All school children were tested regularly.

Dr. Taylor told me that if the tuberculin tests on my children were still negative when they reached sixteen, then I could relax. If they got tuberculosis after that, they would be picking it up from restaurants, sidewalks, and the wide, wide world, but no longer from me.

Old Disease, New Victims

TWELVE

When I started writing this book in late 1990, my daughter Judy, an artist in Santa Barbara, California, said she would help edit and typeset the book for publication. She suddenly seemed to sprout tuberculosis antennae.

Letters began to arrive with clippings from the *Santa Barbara News-Press* and *Los Angeles Times* newspapers. First her local paper issued a screaming headline on February 25, 1991: "County in grip of TB epidemic; Latinos hard hit." The article stated that 81 cases appeared in 1990, a disease rate 100% higher than in 1989. The outbreak is statewide, with an average of 14.5 victims per 100,000 population, and Santa Barbara's "epidemic" rate is 22%. Records show that 78% of the 1990 TB victims were foreign born. Latinos accounted for 70% of the cases; Asian and Pacific Islanders, 14%; whites, 16 percent. Twenty-six percent of the foreign-born victims arrived in the U.S. less than a year ago. Of all cases, 36% were children.

The article went on to state that since September, 1,522 residents of Santa Barbara County had undergone TB skin tests. Of those, 421 showed a positive reaction. Those testing positive are undergoing preventative treatment, according to Dr. Alan Chovil, chief of the county preventative diseases services. Most of these people are friends, co-workers or family members in close contact with victims of the disease.

The new cases are turning up primarily at medical screenings for children entering school or during county immunization clinics. Hospital emergency rooms have been seeing an increasing number of walk-in patients who are very ill.

Health officials recommended caution for parents who employ "nannies" or unlicensed day care who are foreign born. They suggest parents require TB tests of such child-care providers. They further recommend that elderly, unlicensed babysitters with chronic coughs also be tested, "because TB was common decades ago and can lie dormant for many years." Licensed child-care providers, school and medical personnel are routinely screened for TB, the officials said.

They add that actively suffering TB victims get a series of drugs daily for six to nine months. The treatment renders patients virtually non-communicable within days. A preventative drug known as INH is given daily for six months to people testing positive for dormant bacteria. The medicines will stop the disease, but the health officials said that the treatments had to be closely monitored as many people tend to stop taking the pills. "They forget, or they feel fine and don't think it important."

This latter situation has been one of the major problems with Third World treatment of the disease. When the pills have to be taken for so many months, people slough off. Consequently, TB teams have to ride herd on the pill-takers, and rarely do they have the manpower to do a thorough job.

Every newspaper clipping Judy sent presented a new detail of today's TB problems. In the Santa Barbara *Independent,* for instance, in an earlier January 31, 1991, article on the same subject, the reporter stated that Dr. Chovil associated the rise in TB cases to the 1986 Simpson-Mazzoli Immigration Reform and Control Act, commonly known as the amnesty bill, which severely limited employment opportunities for illegal immigrants. The article also mentioned that for each of the 81 active TB cases in the county, "some 20 to 50 of the patients' associates—co-workers, roommates, and relatives—were contacted by the county health department and treated preventatively ...Because the antibiotics can be hard on the liver, people over 35 are generally treated only if they come down with an active infection."

The account from the *Los Angeles Times* , May 14, 1991, was glum. "Los Angeles County is failing in its efforts to control its growing tuberculosis epidemic... The county's tuberculosis rate has risen since 1988 to more than 2½ times the national average—an increase traced largely to immigration, homelessness and the spread of the AIDS virus, which leaves infected people especially vulnerable to tuberculosis.

"The rate, 24.1 cases per 100,000 people, is the highest seen here since the advent of modern drugs to prevent and treat tuberculosis."

The article claims that TB rates are also alarmingly high in San Francisco, Oakland, Long Beach, Newark, New York and Miami.

Efforts to control the epidemic in Los Angeles are failing, according to the article, due to shortages of manpower and money. It ends with a statement from Dr. Wilbur Y. Hallett, a pulmonary disease specialist in Glendale and a member of the lung association board, "[The county supervisors] may feel, 'What the heck, it's not as bad as AIDS, maternal health, something like that. We want to try and convince them that if we don't do something, it will become that bad."

Not to be outdone by our California correspondent, my husband plucked a small article out of our own *Des Moines Register,* on February 17, 1991. This one said that federal tuberculosis officials reported possibly the worst TB increase on record in 1990. Even more distressing, they say, is the appearance of a strain of the disease that is resistant to anti-TB drugs.

The 1990 U.S. tuberculosis count stands at 23,720, with a thousand or more case reports still likely to come in. "The HIV virus that causes AIDS has triggered a TB turnaround," officials stated.

And then I found a similar but amplified article in the rural *CappersWeekly* newspaper, which I subscribe to because they occasionally print the verses I still am writing in my eighties. This article from April 23, 1991, quotes Dixie Snider, chief of the TB division at the Centers for Disease Control in Atlanta. "It's obviously disturbing," Snider says. "It's completely unprecedented in what tuberculosis has actually been doing since the last century." What TB has been doing, till now, was going down. And now suddenly, it's going up again, fast.

Adding to the problem, Snider said, is the apparent increase in drug-resistant TB. A Miami hospital reported 29 drug-resistant TB cases last year, and that number is growing. "That's the most disturbing thing that's happened," Snider said. "If they take over and become a significant part of the pool of tuberculosis organisms that are out there, our whole strategy for TB treatment and prevention has got to be completely revised."

Judy found another headline story in the July 6, 1991, *Santa Barbara News-Press*. "County tuberculosis cases jump 30%," it read. Dr. Chovil was quoted again, "It's serious because we are getting more people infected within the county. We are building a reservoir of disease that will haunt us for 50 or 60 years."

Latinos are hardest hit, representing 67% of the 40 new cases reported during the first four months of the year. County Health Officer Dr. Sarah Miller said many people with the disease bring it from Mexico, where it is relatively uncontrolled.

Dr. Miller adds that many of the infected are former residents of a small village in the Mexican state of Oaxaca, who now live in Santa Maria in the northern part of Santa Barbara County.

The doctors are particularly concerned about the infection of U.S.-born children with the disease. Dr. Chovil explained that because nine out of ten people with TB never become ill but still carry the disease, tuberculosis outbreaks are likely to continue for at least sixty years. Old age, a weakened immune system and other health problems can bring on the acute reinfection phase of the disease in later life. "You can be infectious a long time before getting sick," he said.

"Protection has to come from a TB program" of tracking victims and their contacts and providing them with treatment and immunization. The county has hired additional staff to beef up such a program for the Santa Barbara area.

The newspapers paint a grim picture. After reading them all, Judy reported that she had decided it was time to get a TB test. "I hadn't been tested since I left high school," she wrote. "I was probably tested in 1967 when I taught a year in Germany, but I'm not really certain. I went over to a neighborhood clinic and had the test done. It's certainly easy. The nurse just slid a thin needle under the skin on my forearm and squeezed a bit of solution in. She put a Band-Aid over the spot and told me to come back within 48 to 72 hours. She gave me the paper insert that was with the test material, and it is labeled 'Tuberculin Purified Protein Derivative (Mantoux).' "

That appears to be the same TB test that has been of critical importance all these years in identifying the primary infection.

"I kept peeking under the bandage," Judy went on. "But nothing happened. I went back and showed the nurses my non-reacting arm, and that was that. Still negative after all these years."

We assume that our other daughter, a computer engineer in Kansas City, is just as healthy, though she hasn't bothered to retest.

When TB is caught today, it can usually be cured, or at least chemically controlled. But it's not easy for either the doctors or the patients. It takes discipline, vigilance and constant care. We owe it to future generations to continue the battle against tuberculosis everywhere on this planet. The colorful little stamps I first saw in second grade helped tremendously to decimate the disease. Perhaps we need imaginative programs like that again. We need to make certain that when our children rocket to outer space to start new civilizations, there will be no tuberculosis bacterium among those 21st century Adams and Eves.

One Last Song

THIRTEEN

My life has been a story of tuberculosis ever since my Grandma Cherry took my sister Mary on her knee and fed her from her spoon.

Mary died from tuberculosis, followed by my baby brother Arnold and then my mother. My remaining sister and one of my brothers suffered minor outbreaks but survived to old age. I had four hemorrhages and spent more than three years in a TB sanatorium. But my own children are free of tuberculosis and do not have to live with the memories that sift through my mind.

My own experience with tuberculosis was physically painless. For me it meant disappointments and setbacks of my plans. Yet I have seen and heard the suffering of advanced cases. I have watched them struggle for breath. I have heard their coughs. I have seen the horrible contents of sputum cups at each bedside and heard during interminable nights the continual coughing and spitting in the darkness.

I watched my own mother suffer when her throat was so ravaged she could no longer swallow any food but a raw egg. I can only imagine the frustration and sorrow she had to bear the six long years she spent in bed, unable to take part in family activities. After baby Arnold died, we could never coax our mother to sing with us again.

I remember one night when I was sleeping in my mother's room. The house was silent except for her coughing. Suddenly I awoke to her soft voice singing an old gospel hymn.

There were ninety and nine that safely lay
In the shelter of the fold,
But one was out on the hills away
Far off from the gates of gold.

Out in the desert He heard its cry
So sick and helpless and ready to die.
None knew how deep the waters He crossed
Ere the Shepherd found His sheep that was lost.

I lay there trembling as she sang. I thought she'd died and gone to heaven. When I finally asked if she was all right, she said she knew everyone was asleep, but she just felt like singing, so she did.

She didn't sing for happiness as in earlier and better days. She was herself that poor lost lamb. None of us could help her then. Today it is possible to find all the lost lambs of the world and care for them, if we will.

What We Need to Know

The greatest tuberculosis danger today is complacency and lack of knowledge. Too many people think that TB is a rare disease now, and that modern drugs will cure it, so why worry.

It is rapidly becoming a less-than-rare disease in this country. And it was not the use of modern anti-tuberculosis drugs that brought the disease to its knees in the 1940s. It was a pervasive team operation among health professionals all over the country which for decades efficiently identified active carriers and isolated them in sanatoria, rapidly reducing the active sources of contamination within the general population, while teaching families how to prevent further infection. The drugs only arrived at the tail end of this magnificent medical achievement, essentially replacing the sanatoria.

Today we have the drugs, but due to the near-eradication of the disease since the 1950s, the formerly vast network of TB health professionals has diminished and is rusty, under-staffed, and minimally funded. The sanatoria are gone, their records often destroyed. The National Tuberculosis Association has changed its name to the American Lung Association and has turned much of its energy and funds to asthma and the dangers of smoking. We are already seeing the result—the beginnings of a rampant epidemic in a public that is as fully ignorant of the ways of tuberculosis as my parents' and grandparents' generations were.

What do we need once more to know? I will try to simplify and summarize here what I have learned.

WHAT IS TUBERCULOSIS? It is a disease caused by a

bacterium, *Mycobacterium tuberculosis.* There are two phases to the disease. The first or primary phase, usually occurring in early childhood, is the entry of the bacteria into the body. Usually the body's natural strength will encase the bacteria in protective tubercles. Tubercles are formed wherever the bacteria locate in the body but most often in the lungs. The tubercles will, in the majority of cases, remain intact and thus noninfectious. The second or reinfection phase begins when the walls of the tubercles break down, releasing the captive bacilli into the body. The bacilli may attack any organ, bone or membrane of the body, but often concentrate in the lungs. If the reinfection phase causes illness and death, it is called acute. If the reinfection phase is minor and of a relapsing nature, it is called chronic. The acute phase often strikes infants and young adults; the chronic phase may last into old age. Victims of both the acute and chronic reinfection phases can spread the bacteria to those around them.

HOW IS THE BACTERIA SPREAD? It is an airborne bacteria, riding on dust and moisture particles. The source of the bacteria is primarily the sputum or saliva of an infected person, but feces and other body fluids may also carry the disease. The bacteria can be transferred in many ways. Simply being within twenty feet of an infected person who is coughing or spitting is sufficient. Touching or kissing an infected person and handling objects or clothing they have used may transfer the disease. Eating from silverware, plates and cups used by an infected person can be a source of contamination. Handling shoes that have stepped in sputum on the sidewalk or street can transfer the bacteria. The disease can also be spread from TB-infected cattle, directly from handling them or from drinking infected raw milk and from eating infected rare beef.

HOW DOES ONE DETECT PRIMARY TUBERCULOSIS? The primary phase of tuberculosis can only be detected through the tuberculin test, commonly called the TB skin test. A positive test reaction means the person has the primary TB infection, though he or she may appear in robust health and show no signs whatever of illness.

HOW IS THE PRIMARY PHASE TREATED? Most people who test positive do not develop the acute reinfection phase, but the potential is always there. Anyone who tests positive needs to follow a doctor's advice and may be asked to take a six-month series of INH (isoniazid) pills to kill the bacteria. If reactors do not take the pills, they should have periodic X-rays the rest of their lives to check for any emergence of the dormant bacteria and should be extremely careful about colds and coughs.

HOW IS THE ACUTE PHASE DETECTED? If the disease progresses from primary to acute reinfection phase, there can be many symptoms in addition to a positive tuberculin test. The most common symptoms are a deep, chesty cough with mucous, fever, and a general wasting away of the body, extreme thinness, weakness and fatigue. Occasionally, when the lungs are infected, a hemorrhage will bring up blood from coughing. Tuberculosis affects other parts of the body than the lungs and can attack the spine and other bones and membranes. The acute phase, untreated, can result in a painful death. The most common age for acute reinfection is that of young adulthood.

HOW IS THE ACUTE PHASE TREATED? The primary anti-tuberculosis drugs in use today are isoniazid, rifampin, PZA and ethambutol. If the drugs are taken as prescribed, daily over a period of six to twelve months, they are extremely effective. Usually a combination of three of these is used for the first two months of treatment, in case bacteria are resistant to one or more. Some new strains of TB have been reported, however, that are not reacting to any of these drugs. Prior to the use of these drugs the only treatment was bedrest (often two or three years), good nutrition and several types of lung surgery.

HOW IS THE CHRONIC PHASE DETECTED? It is a phase that is often not detected because the infected person is not seriously ill and usually has only a persistent, minor cough or throat inflammation. The chronic tuberculosis carrier may be an older person, if not elderly, and is a particularly dangerous source of infection to extended families.

HOW IS CHRONIC TB TREATED? If it is found, it is treated the same as acute tuberculosis, with antibiotics.

WHAT ABOUT AIDS AND TUBERCULOSIS? The person infected with the HIV virus may be more than ordinarily subject to tuberculosis. The HIV virus can develop over time into AIDS, which is a syndrome of auto-immune deficient diseases, most of them terminal. One of them is tuberculosis. If the HIV infected person also is infected with the TB bacteria, the body may not be able to rally enough strength to form tubercles to encase the bacteria. Thus the bacteria could advance rapidly to the acute tuberculosis phase and kill the host.

WHAT ABOUT PREVENTION AND TREATMENT? The same advice on prevention of TB in the general population goes for HIV infected persons as well, and even more so. It is important for the infected person to be well-rested, to eat well and to avoid situations that might result in contact with TB germs. If acute TB takes over, the body is often too weak and wasted to respond well to anti-tuberculosis drugs.

WHAT IS THE WORLD TB SITUATION? TB has been phenomenally decreased in the United States, Canada, western Europe and other areas that have strong modern health care systems. It is still rampant in the Third World, however, where two-thirds of the people of this earth reside. It will never be eradicated until several generations of children (and cattle) all over the world have lived through their spans of life without infection. Drugs cannot accomplish that, only prevention and knowledge.

HOW CAN I PROTECT MY FAMILY AND MYSELF?

1. Recognize tuberculosis as a present danger. Be aware that carriers can be anywhere, but especially within poor, immigrant populations living in crowded conditions with poor sanitation and nutrition. Help to change that wherever you can.

2. Be sure that your children's schools and day-care centers are licensed and that all staff are TB-tested.

3. Support TB testing of children within the schools.

4. If you hire babysitters or household help who are foreign-born or elderly, be sure they are TB-tested. Be especially wary of someone who is very thin and has a persistent cough.

5. Practice good sanitation and proper table manners at home and in restaurants.

6. Wash hands with hot water and soap before eating, both at home and at restaurants. Wash your hands frequently during your day's activities.

7. Never drink from the same glass, cup, bottle or can as another person. Forbid your children to do so. Wash or at least

wipe off the tops of bottles and cans before drinking from them. Use clean paper or styrofoam cups whenever possible. Consider the potential contamination of communion chalices.

8. Never share eating utensils with another person.

9. Use serving spoons to dip from a bowl of food to individual plates, and a butter knife to distribute butter. Do not lick a knife and then reach for more butter with it. Do not use your fork or spoon to take a helping from the serving dish.

10. Wash your dishes carefully, using detergent and hot water. Rinse in hot water. A dash of Chlorox in the rinse water will help kill germs. Air dry your dishes or be sure your dishtowels are clean. Use an electric dishwasher if possible.

11. Be sure that dishwashing facilities for schools and organizations are sanitary and that people who wash dishes for groups use clean, hot, soapy water, changed often. Wellmeaning community organizations who serve fund-raising suppers may not have sanitation uppermost on their minds.

12. Buy only pasteurized milk products. Health food stores offer raw milk products from herds they claim are TB tested. One infected cow that escapes testing can quickly infect the entire herd. There is nothing "unnatural" about pasteurized milk. It only means that it has been heated to kill bacteria.

13. Ask the management of your favorite restaurant if their food handlers are routinely TB-tested. Is the dishwashing properly handled so that tableware is sterilized? Keep them on their toes.

14. Keep kitchen and bathroom areas clean and neat, especially when several people are sharing them.

15. Wash your hands after handling the soles of your shoes. Shoes pick up TB bacilli from the street where people have spit. Avoid going barefoot along city streets and sidewalks.

16. Cover your mouth when you cough, and ask others to do so. Use paper tissues instead of handkerchiefs.

17. Take care of colds. Go to bed and rest. Gargle with salt water or antiseptic mouthwash and wash your hands carefully. Avoid children with colds.

18. If you or your children partake in group sports, watch to be sure a coach doesn't pass a communal water bottle among participants. Be sure coaches understand the reasons for sanitation in group situations.

19. Likewise, don't share communal towels used to wipe sweat from players' bodies.

20. If you travel in Mexico, Asia and other Third World nations, be extremely careful about cleanliness and food handling. Be aware of the potential for air-borne contamination when traveling in close quarters with people who are coughing or spitting. In Mexico, beware of raw milk. Most Mexican dairies and processing plants are modern and sanitary, and pasteurized milk products can be found almost everywhere, but occasionally in small towns and markets, you may run into local raw milk, butter, yogurt or cheese products that are not *pasteurizada*. Oaxaca cheese has generally been cooked, but ranch cheeses are uncooked, thus not pasteurized. Raw milk purchased in the markets can be pasteurized by bringing it slowly to a boil, stirring constantly to avoid scorching.

21. Keep strong and healthy with good food, exercise and rest. When you attempt to eliminate cholesterol from your diet, bear in mind that TB patients in the past were fed a diet rich in eggs, butter, cream and milk to help their bodies build calcium walls around tubercle bacilli.

22. Reflect on this: the extremely thin physique popular in women's magazines today is the exact image of the tubercular body.

SOURCES

Most of the factual information on tuberculosis interwoven throughout this narrative comes from two important books written by one man, Dr. Jay Arthur Myers of Minnesota. The first one is entitled *Tuberculosis: A Half Century of Study and Conquest.* The second is *Captain of All These Men of Death: Tuberculosis Historical Highlights.* The former was published in 1970, the latter in 1977, both by Warren H. Green, Inc., 8356 Olive Boulevard, St. Louis, Missouri 63132. These are fascinating books full of an enormous amount of historical and research data, concisely and compassionately written by a clinician who has observed, studied and worked with tuberculosis for more than half a century.

A partial list of other books on the subject include:

1. Bryder, Linda. *Below the magic mountain: a social history of tuberculosis in twentieth-century Britain,* Oxford: Clarendon Press; New York: Oxford University Press, 1988.
2. Caldwell, Mark. *The Last Crusade: the War on Consumption,* New York: Atheneum, 1988.
3. Cummins, S. Lyle. *Tuberculosis in History, from the 17th century to our own times,* Baltimore: Williams and Wilkins, 1949.
4. Davis, Lenwood G., *A history of tuberculosis in the black community: a working bibliography,* Monticello, Ill.: Council of Planning Librarians, 1975.
5. Mann, Thomas (trans. H. T. Lowe-Porter), *The Magic Mountain,* New York: Vintage Books, 1969
6. Meachen, G. Norman. *A Short History of Tuberculosis,* London: John Bale, Sons & Danielsson Ltd., 1936.
7. Paterson, Elizabeth M. *History of the National Conference of Tuberculosis Workers: 1090–1955,* New York: National Tuberculosis Association, c1956.
8. Sattler, Eric E. *A History of Tuberculosis from the time of Sylvius to the present day,* Cincinnati: R. Clarke & Co., 1883.
9. Sontag, Susan. Illness as Metaphor and AIDS and Its Metaphors, New York: Doubleday, Anchor edition, 1990.
10. Teller, Michael E. *The tuberculosis movement: a public*

health campaign in the progressive era, New York: Greenwood Press, 1988.
11. Wilson, Julius Lane. *Early tuberculosis sanatoria in the United States and Canada*, Santa Fe: (n.p.) , 1969.

Thanks to Ventura County Historical Society Librarian Charles Johnson for helping to compile this short bibliography.

The information about milk in Mexico in Chapter 12 is from Carl Franz' *The People's Guide to Mexico*, Santa Fe: John Muir Publications, 1986.

ACKNOWLEDGEMENTS

We deeply appreciate the editing help given by Barbara Tompkins, typographical advice from Roger Levenson, darkroom work on the cover photo by Bill Dewey and consultation on medical aspects of the book from Dr. Alan Chovil, Santa Barbara County Preventative Diseases Services.

The typeface used in this book is Claire De Lune, designed
by Judith Sutcliffe: The Electric Typographer. Type was set
on a Macintosh and output on a LaserWriter Plus.
Book designed by Judith Sutcliffe.